AIR
AMBULANCE

© Haynes Publishing 2019

First published in September 2019

A catalogue record for this book is available from the British Library.

ISBN 978 1 78521 206 2

Library of Congress control no. 2018938907

Published by Haynes Publishing,
Sparkford, Yeovil, Somerset BA22 7JJ, UK.
Tel: 01963 440635
Int. tel: +44 1963 440635
Website: www.haynes.com

Haynes North America Inc.,
859 Lawrence Drive, Newbury Park,
California 91320, USA.

Printed in Malaysia.

Air Ambulances UK

Air Ambulances UK is the official national charity which supports the lifesaving work of the nation's 21 air ambulance charities by creating fundraising partnerships with nationwide businesses, organisations, trusts and foundations and major donors.

The funds raised help air ambulance charities to collectively make around 70 lifesaving missions every day across the UK and remain the world-leaders in Helicopter Emergency Medical Service provision. Registered Charity Number: 1161153
www.airambulancesuk.org

AIR AMBULANCE

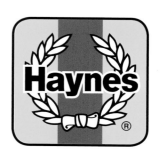

Operations Manual

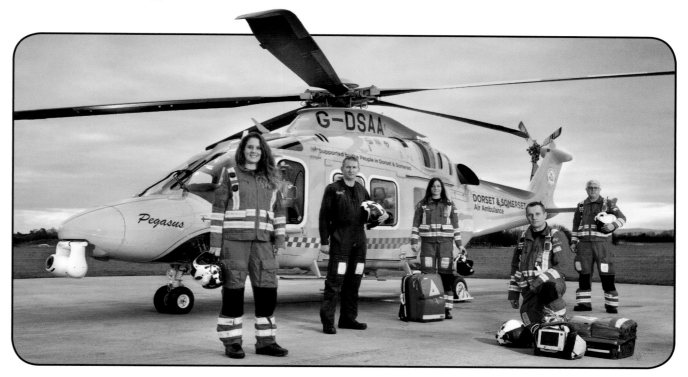

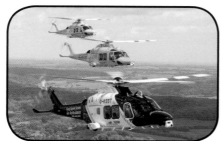

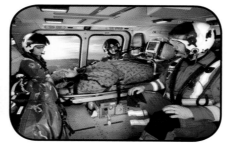

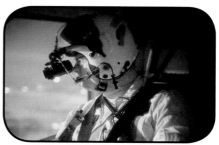

An insight into the role and operation of helicopter air ambulances in the UK

Claire Robinson

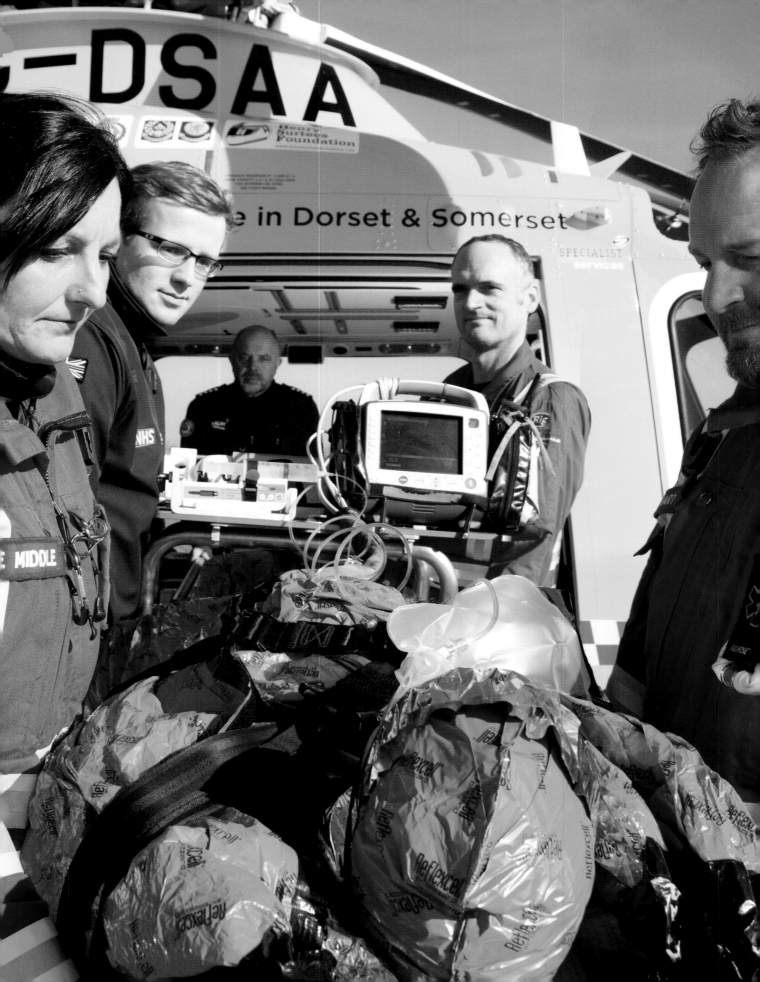

Contents

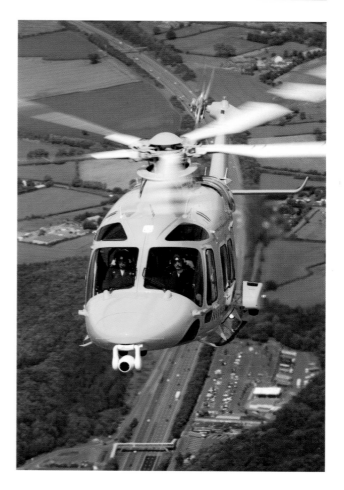

RIGHT The Leonardo AW169 helicopter is now in widespread use with UK air ambulance services.
(Leonardo Helicopters/Simon Pryor)

OPPOSITE The critical care team transfers a casualty to the DSAA helicopter. *(Leonardo Helicopters/Simon Pryor)*

Foreword

by Jenson Button

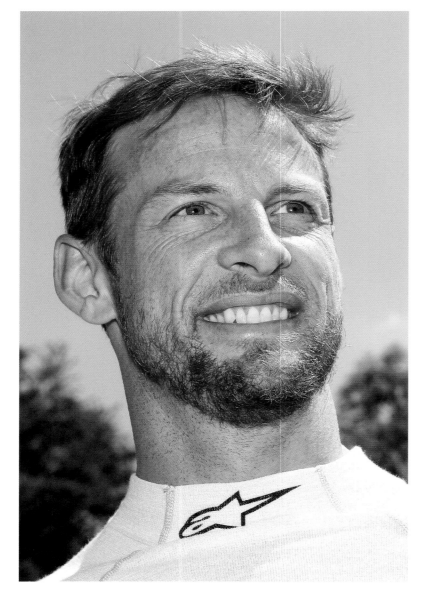

I have been vice-patron and ambassador of Dorset and Somerset Air Ambulance (DSAA) since its formation in 2000, so I was delighted to be asked to write a foreword to the first-ever Haynes Manual on air ambulances.

Coming from the fast, dangerous and high-pressure sport of motor racing, I understand the importance of having a highly skilled, hard-working and dedicated team behind you. The crews of every air ambulance service across the UK help to save thousands of people every year and this excellent manual provides a comprehensive insight into the important, life-saving work that goes on behind the scenes.

I was born in Frome, Somerset, a rural part of the county serviced by DSAA, and I regularly saw first-hand its importance to the local community. Critically ill or injured patients across the two counties can have a world-class clinical team by their side within a matter of minutes, brought to them by one of DSAA's experienced and skilled pilots.

When every second counts, having cutting-edge technology to support you is crucial. DSAA's AW169 helicopter (whose manufacturer, Leonardo, has its UK base in Yeovil) is a state-of-the-art aircraft, fully fitted out with the latest medical equipment and having the range to fly back-to-back missions if need be.

Of course, none of this would be possible without the support of the public. Air ambulances across the UK are funded by charitable donations – and every little helps.

Striving for excellence takes dedication, commitment and enthusiasm. When this is backed up with passionate supporters it creates something very special. I hope you enjoy reading this manual and consider showing your support to your local air ambulance – you never know when you might need them.

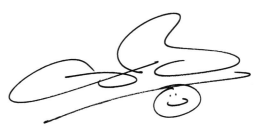

Jenson Button

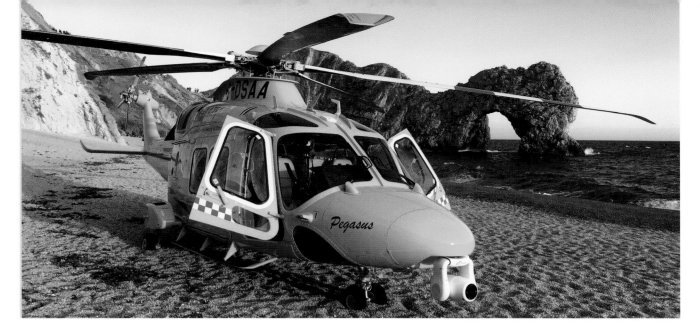

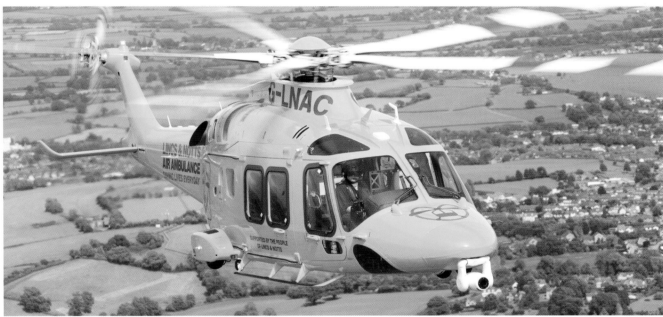

TOP Air ambulances enable medical teams to reach a casualty as quickly as possible, bringing the hospital to the patient, particularly in locations which would be inaccessible by any other means. *(Leonardo Helicopters/Simon Pryor)*

ABOVE Charitable donations from companies, organisations and the public keep the UK's air ambulances flying. *(Leonardo Helicopters/Simon Pryor)*

RIGHT Each air ambulance service has a highly skilled, dedicated crew of clinicians and pilots. Here, a patient arrives at London's Air Ambulance helipad at the Royal London Hospital. *(London's Air Ambulance)*

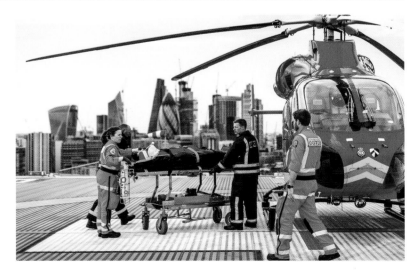

Introduction

Most people in the UK will think they have some concept of what an air ambulance is: they will be familiar with the sight of the helicopters and the name itself seems self-explanatory. In reality, there is much more to it than the uninitiated would expect.

The most common assumption is that the function of an air ambulance is the same as a regular ambulance, just using a different mode of transport. In the beginning, this was partly true but over the last 30 or more years, air ambulance services have evolved beyond recognition. Now, the focus is on bringing critical care directly to the patient wherever they may be and, if necessary, performing life-saving surgery in situ. The remit and capabilities of the air ambulance medical teams often go beyond the role of paramedics in road ambulances. In many cases, the procedures some air ambulance crews can carry out will only be encountered in critical care units in hospitals.

The image of the helicopter airlifting the patient to hospital also fails to tell the whole story. When circumstances demand it, the air ambulance clinicians might arrive by car or even motorcycle. Even if they arrive by air, the move of the patient to hospital might still be by land ambulance but accompanied by the air ambulance crew.

Probably the most common misconception – and one that is at the heart of its idiosyncratic features – is that the service is not part of the NHS. The different regional air ambulances are, all but one, run independently by discrete charities. A typical reaction to this is surprise or even outrage that the government doesn't support this essential life-saving service. However, it will become apparent over the course of this publication that this is not the case and that the charity funding model has fostered innovation and enabled the air ambulance service to develop in ways that wouldn't have been possible within the public sector.

There is a fundamental difference in approach between the air ambulance charities and the NHS. The NHS is entrusted with

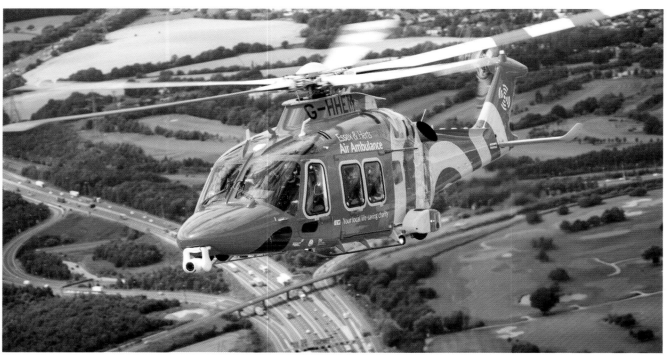

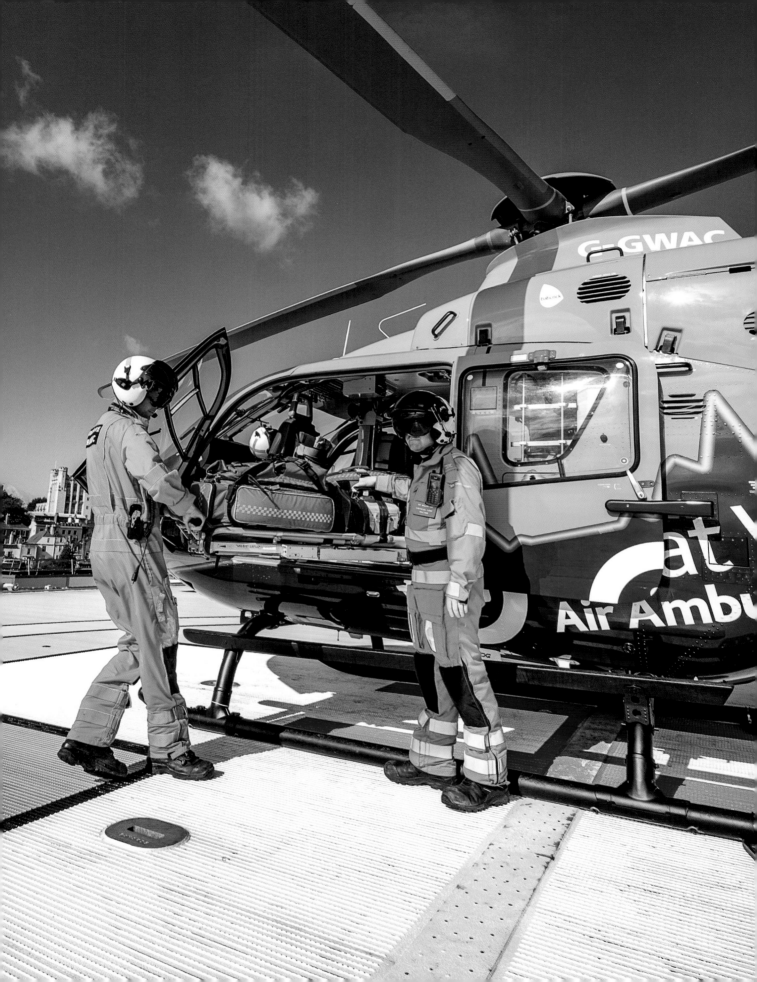

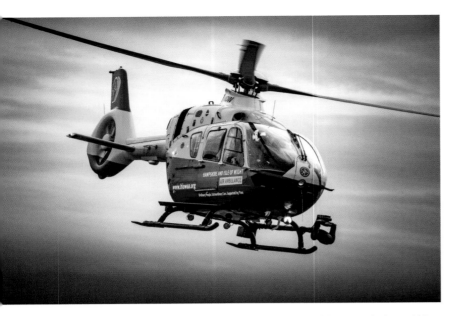

ABOVE Hampshire
and Isle of Wight Air
Ambulance's Airbus
H135 helicopter can
carry three or four
crew members.
(Simon Heron)

helping those that might not receive treatment
quickly enough otherwise. And as long as
they can convince the charity-giving public to
support them, this is what they do.

Another feature of the charity set-up is that
each air ambulance organisation operates in
its own individual way, using different types of
helicopters, crew arrangements and ways of
working with the NHS – each tailored to their
local geography and population. This variety
has the added benefit that all services can
observe and gain from each other's experience
as they attempt to tackle new situations and
deploy new techniques and technologies. The
progress and innovation achieved by the air
ambulance service has been phenomenal and
their medicine is groundbreaking, spawning
a new medical sub-specialty: Pre-Hospital
Emergency Medicine.

This might be giving the impression of
competition between the air ambulance and the
NHS but nothing could be further from the truth.
In most cases the medical staff are in fact NHS
employees but part-funded by the charities, and
the air ambulance service works seamlessly with
the NHS hospitals. The air ambulance service
has a healthy symbiotic relationship with the
NHS and innovations pass in both directions.

looking after the health of the population within
a fixed budget. Everything must be approached
on a cost-benefit basis, attempting to calculate
where each pound will make the most positive
impact. Inevitably, the population becomes
statistics and people who fall ill at the wrong
time or in the wrong place end up becoming
casualties. The air ambulance can approach the
situation from the opposite direction, focused
on the individual rather than the population and

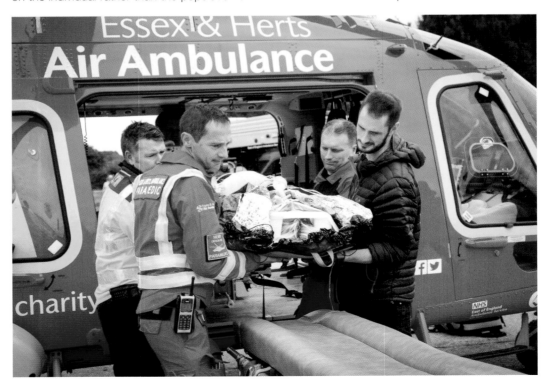

RIGHT Essex & Herts
Air Ambulance is
currently working
towards providing a
full 24/7 operation.
*(Leonardo Helicopters/
Simon Pryor)*

Acknowledgements

At a time when many of us wonder what the purpose or value is in what we do, the air ambulance stands in bright contrast – the crews know that their actions save lives and this is reflected in the passion and dedication they show for their work. Writing this publication has involved countless interviews: talking to the air ambulance teams has been an immense pleasure and in no small part, humbling. I have many people to thank for their time and help.

When Haynes approached Dorset and Somerset Air Ambulance (DSAA), the service chosen as the case study for this book, CEO Bill Sivewright and Communications Manager Tracy Bartram embraced the project from the start and helped drive it forward. Bill's former role as chairman of the Association of Air Ambulances also prompted the wider examination of the air ambulance situation across the UK. Bill and Tracy's practical support, enthusiasm and sense of humour throughout the entire process has been invaluable.

I am particularly grateful to Phil Hyde, DSAA Medical Lead and Paul Owen, DSAA Operational Lead for sharing their insights and giving so generously of their time. Thanks also go to the following DSAA crew members and staff for the time spent talking to me: Claire Baker, Neil Bizzell, Wayne Busby, Mario Carretta, Kirsty Caswell, Emily Cooper, Caroline Guy, Owen Hammett, Max Hoskins, Farhad Islam (Izzy), Dan Kitteridge, Phil Merritt, Ian Mew, Jonny Price, Matt Sawyer and Michelle Walker. Paul Holmes at South Western Ambulance Service Foundation Trust (SWASFT) was also very helpful in explaining the processes of Helicopter Emergency Medical Service (HEMS) dispatch.

Gareth Davies and Roderick Mackenzie provided valuable insight and information on the workings of London's Air Ambulance and the history of pre-hospital emergency medicine (PHEM) respectively. Geoff Newman was extremely generous in sharing his memories (and photographs) of the very first UK air ambulance, which he helped to found in Cornwall in 1987. Thanks also to Andrew Scriven at the Association of Air Ambulances for filling in any historical gaps.

When it came to writing about the AW169, Geoff Russell and Jim Griffin at Leonardo, and Jan-Marc Van Dam at Specialist Aviation Services, were very helpful. Special mention should be made of Leonardo photographer Simon Pryor, who shot many of the wonderful images you will see in these pages.

Steve Rendle, my editor at Haynes, was enthusiastic, patient, helpful and flexible from day one and didn't even fall off his chair when I announced I was unexpectedly pregnant halfway through the writing process!

Finally, thanks to my husband, Hugh, for his endless patience and support while I lived and breathed the world of air ambulances for a good many months. And to my children, Daisy and Phoebe, who put up with Mummy hiding behind a computer screen for far too long.

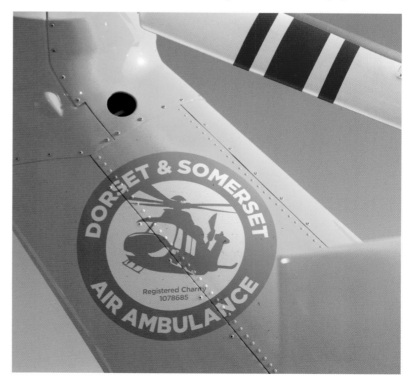

BELOW Many people have given their time freely to contribute to this book, particularly the team at Dorset and Somerset Air Ambulance (DSAA). *(Leonardo Helicopters/ Simon Pryor)*

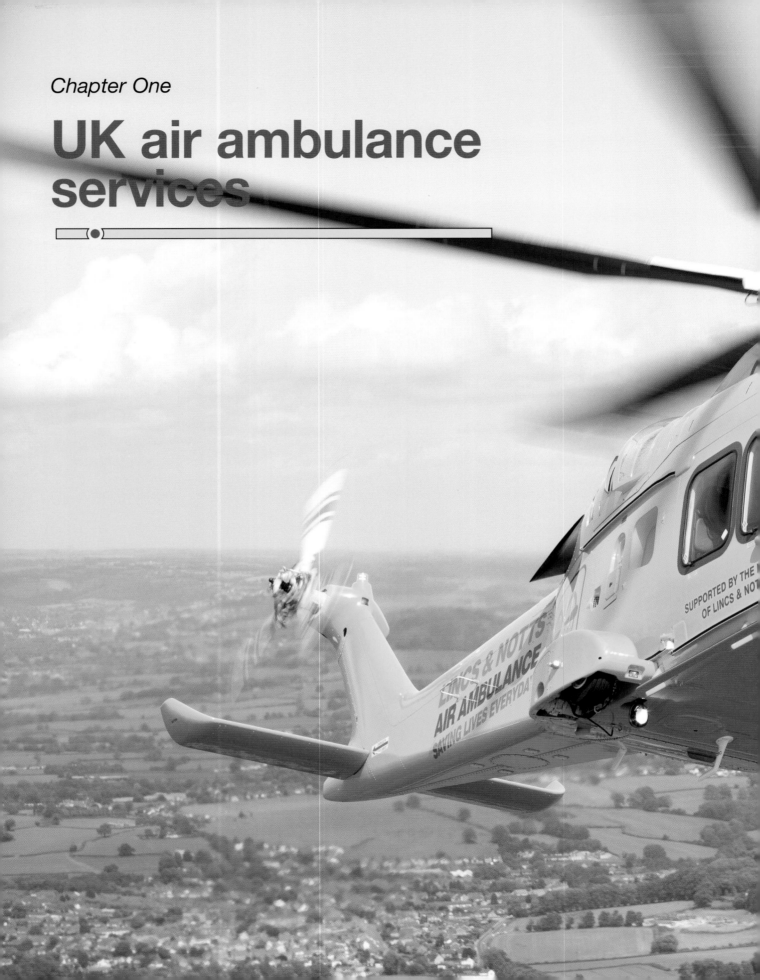

Chapter One

UK air ambulance services

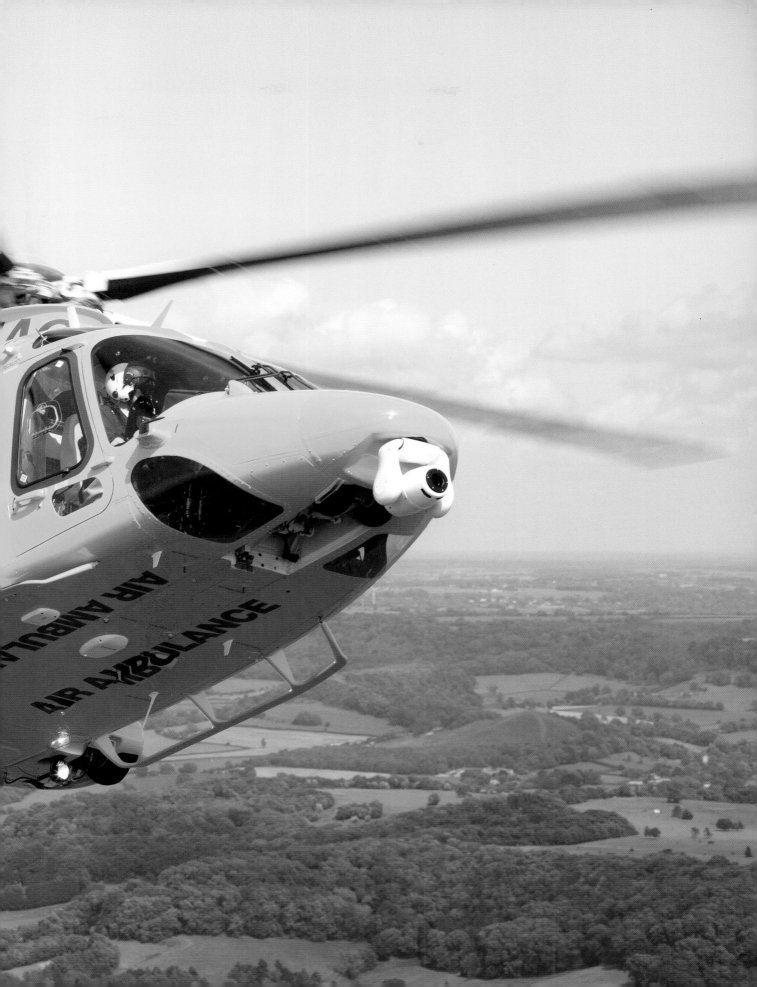

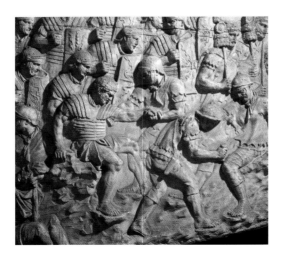

RIGHT Roman soldiers aiding their wounded comrades after a battle against the Dacians, shown in a relief of Trajan's Column, from 2nd century Rome. *(DeAgostini/Getty Images)*

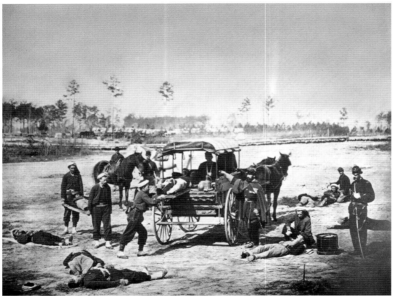

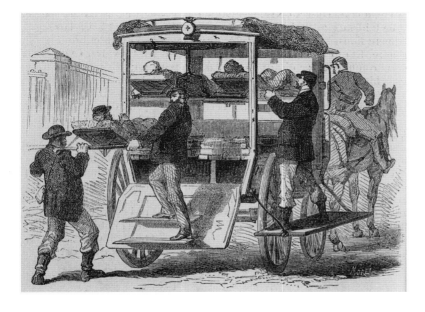

From hammocks to helicopters

The earliest ambulance services were fairly rudimentary affairs. On the battlefields of Roman Britain, teams of riders carried away the wounded on horses, with soldiers earning a piece of gold each time they saved a life. During the Anglo-Saxon period that followed, sick and injured patients of any rank were transported in hammocks or wheeled stretchers known as litters, or carried in carts that were either hand-drawn or pulled by mules.

By the late 19th century, patients were usually delivered to their doctor's surgery or local hospital on litters that were often pushed by police or firefighters, sometimes even by taxi drivers. Horse-drawn ambulances followed, with the first such service starting in Liverpool in 1884 and the last one used in 1912, when four-legged transportation gave way to four-wheeled, motorised methods. During the First World War, injured soldiers were evacuated from the battlefield via air transport, with the first recorded British ambulance flight taking place in 1917 in the Sinai Desert when a soldier in the Imperial Camel Corps was shot in the ankle and flown to hospital in a B.E.2c. The trip, which would normally have taken three days by land, took only 45 minutes to complete – medical evacuation by aircraft during times of war has taken place ever since.

In 1946 in the UK, the National Health Service Act paved the way for the introduction of the NHS, which would be established exactly two years later. Driven by two guiding principles, the NHS promised to deliver a health service that was both available to all and free at the point of use, and part of this commitment

CENTRE Members of the Union Army Ambulance Corps collect the wounded from the battlefield on stretchers and load them into a horse-drawn wagon during the American Civil War, circa 1863. *(Archive Photos/Getty Images)*

LEFT Patients being loaded onto a horse-drawn ambulance in the late 19th century. *(DeAgostini/Getty Images)*

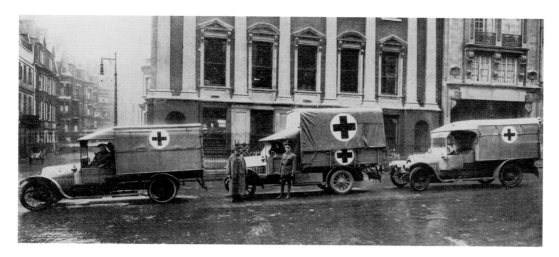

was to make ambulances available for all who needed them.

In those early post-war days, ambulances were essentially just a means of transporting patients. Ambulance staff needed only to have a driving licence and to obtain a certificate in first aid. This remained the case for two decades, until the 1966 Millar report introduced the concept of clinical training for ambulance staff, to enable them to treat a patient as well as transport them.

By 1986, nationwide training schemes were introduced and today's ambulances are crewed by trained emergency medical technicians (EMTs) and paramedics. While both EMTs and paramedics are trained to deal with life-threatening illnesses or injuries, paramedics are also qualified to perform invasive procedures at the scene of an incident, if there is a serious medical emergency.

The UK's ambulance service now comprises 13 individual NHS Ambulance Trusts covering England, Wales, Scotland and Northern Ireland, plus the public ambulance services of the Isle of Man, Guernsey and Jersey (and the British overseas territory of Gibraltar).

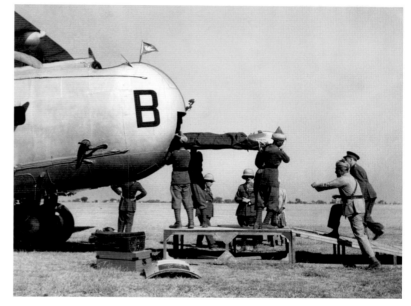

CENTRE Wounded soldiers being airlifted on a British plane during revolts in the North-West Frontier Province, Pakistan, in 1937. *(Heinrich Hoffmann/ullstein bild via Getty Images)*

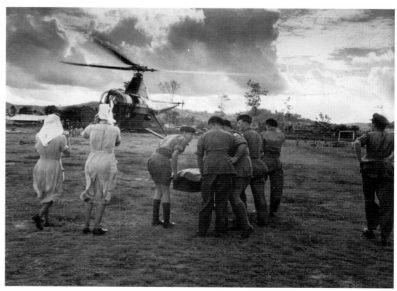

RIGHT A wounded soldier arrives by helicopter at a military hospital in Malaysia, in 1953. *(©Hulton-Deutsch Collection/Corbis via Getty Images)*

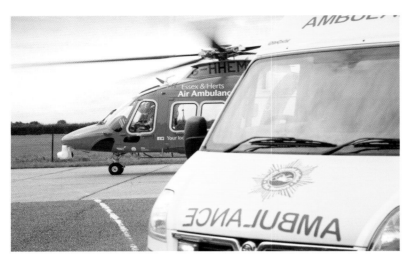

While the coverage provided by these trusts is comprehensive, different geographical regions present different challenges for land-based ambulances: patients may need to be retrieved from remote rural areas, for instance, or from the centre of a busy city at rush hour. At times like these, air ambulances are often a more useful mode of transport and act as an extension of the ambulance service's land vehicles for the transfer of patients to or from hospital.

The helicopters used by air ambulance services have an obvious advantage over ground-based transport of being able to reduce journey time. In the early days of the air ambulance, their superior speed enabled trained medical personnel to be transported to patients quickly and for those patients to be taken from the scene of an incident, packaged up and delivered to hospital faster than would have been possible by road.

These days, however, the main purpose has evolved and the principal role of an air ambulance is to undertake Helicopter Emergency Medical Service (HEMS) missions. This means delivering medical personnel and equipment as close as possible, as rapidly as possible, to the scene of an accident or medical emergency – essentially bringing the hospital to the patient. The patient is then assessed, treated and if further treatment is necessary, airlifted to hospital or sent on by road.

It is widely acknowledged that the speed at which a patient suffering from major trauma is initially treated and delivered to a hospital or trauma facility can significantly affect their chances of survival, as well as the rate and extent of their recovery. This period of time is often called the 'golden hour' and it is used to emphasise the need for urgency in the pre-hospital phase of patient care. Response times are therefore crucial, so reaching these patients and treating them during the golden hour can often mean the difference between life and death.

Helicopters, of course, have their own disadvantages: they can't fly in very bad weather, they face limitations at night, they have space and weight restrictions in terms of what they can carry and, most obviously, they are very expensive. But sometimes they offer the only practical alternative. Our roads are increasingly congested and a growing number of people are participating in outdoor leisure pursuits. Reaching a patient by road and then transporting them to the most appropriate

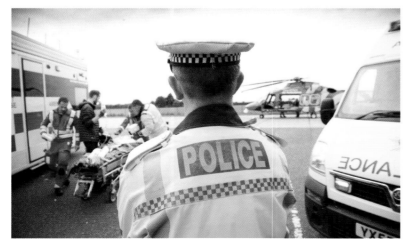

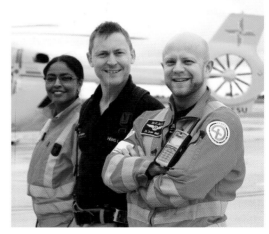

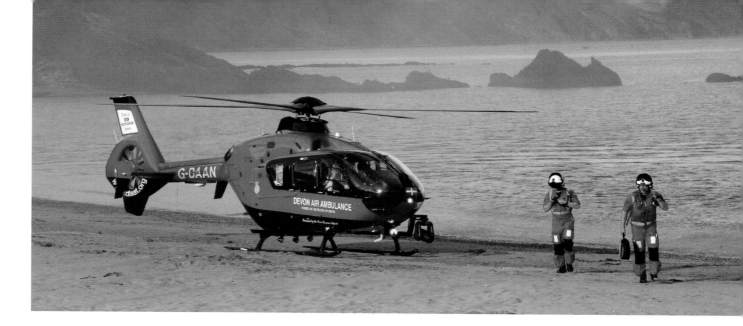

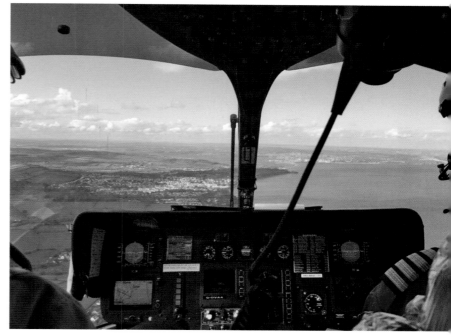

ABOVE Helicopters can reach patients in areas that are difficult to access by road, such as this Devon beach. *(Devon Air Ambulance Trust)*

RIGHT Some ambulance services use a twin-pilot model, while others train their medical staff to act as co-pilots. *(Darren Hall)*

hospital (which is not always the closest one) can be difficult and time-consuming. Far better to bring the clinical team to the patient's side and treat them at the scene of the incident.

Pre-Hospital Emergency Medicine

One of the biggest challenges facing the clinicians on any air ambulance is taking interventions, operations and drugs from the hospital environment out into the street and the workplace and being able to deliver them in a quality-controlled way, when the patient needs them.

In the early days of HEMS, there was initial scepticism and resistance to pre-hospital emergency care procedures from many in the medical community. Pre-Hospital Emergency Medicine (PHEM) wasn't really considered a 'proper' specialty. There was a lot of

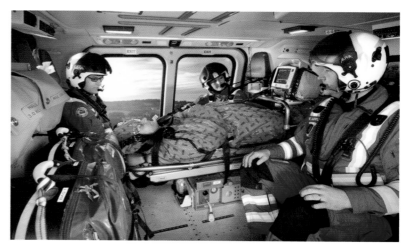

RIGHT If a patient suffering from major trauma is treated and delivered to a hospital during the so-called 'golden hour' their chances are greatly improved. *(Leonardo Helicopters/Simon Pryor)*

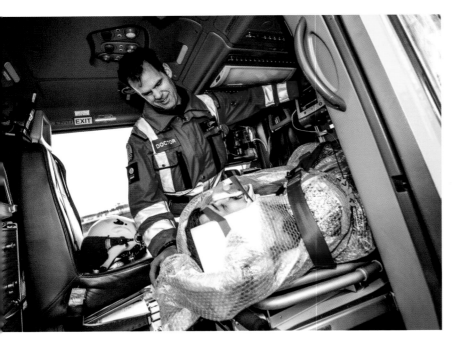

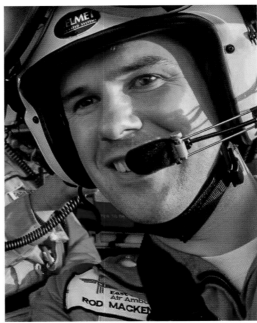

ABOVE In 2011, the General Medical Council accepted the creation of the sub-specialty of Pre-Hospital Emergency Medicine (PHEM). Since then, a number of doctors have been able to train specifically to become consultants in pre-hospital care. *(Hampshire and Isle of Wight Air Ambulance)*

ABOVE RIGHT Roderick Mackenzie, former medical director of Magpas Air Ambulance, is the Faculty of Pre-hospital Care's national PHEM sub-specialty development lead.

apprehension about doctors working in the street, or taking patients away from hospitals. With no recognised training scheme and little or no empirical evidence to show its benefits, pre-hospital care was considered less of an entity by mainstream medicine.

In 2009, the Intercollegiate Board for Training in PHEM (IBTPHEM) was formed. 'In terms of scope of practice, it was recognised that the term "pre-hospital care" covered a very wide range of medical conditions, medical interventions, clinical providers and physical locations,' says Roderick Mackenzie, the Faculty of Pre-Hospital Care's national PHEM sub-specialty development lead and former medical director of Magpas Air Ambulance. Over a ten-year period, Roderick was the principal driving force to develop the IBTPHEM itself and then the sub-specialty. 'It was also recognised that with the evolution of paramedic practice, 99% of pre-hospital care

demand was met, to a high standard, by paramedics,' he says.

IBTPHEM clarified the scope of PHEM practice as 'relating to the underpinning knowledge, technical skills and non-technical (behavioural) skills required to provide safe pre-hospital critical care and safe transfer'. 'Pre-hospital' referred to all environments outside the emergency department, including the scene of the incident, the ambulance and any remote medical facilities. It also related to a particular severity of illness or injury. 'Safe transfer' referred to the process of physically transporting a patient while caring for them in transit.

An extensive curriculum development process, involving the full range of specialties, practitioners and professions, was undertaken to generate the PHEM curriculum framework required to deliver against this scope of practice.

In 2011, the General Medical Council (GMC) accepted the creation of the sub-specialty of PHEM. Since then, it has been recognised that doctors involved in emergency medicine, anaesthesia, intensive care medicine and acute internal medicine are able to train specifically to become consultants in pre-hospital care. A number of consultants have specifically gone through made-to-measure training programmes and are now recognised by the GMC as PHEM-trained doctors – essentially there has been a

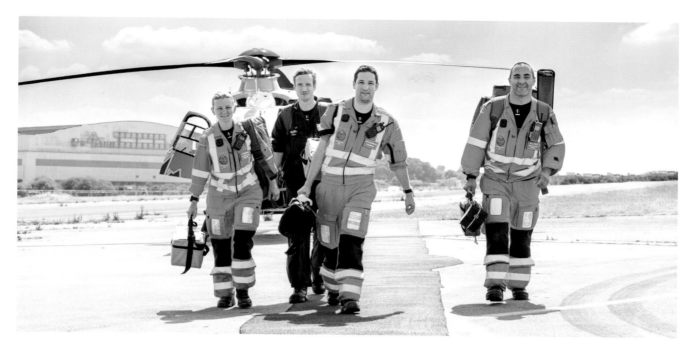

professionalisation of doctors' involvement in pre-hospital care.

'The cross-fertilisation of knowledge between pre-hospital and in-hospital clinicians has changed the understanding of what is and what is not possible for patients in the pre-hospital domain,' says Phil Hyde, Medical Lead at DSAA. 'This has really helped to streamline and improve care for patients.'

'It was the birth of a new star,' says Gareth Davies, medical director of London's Air Ambulance. 'These things don't happen very often in medicine, where a new sub-specialty is created. It's still in its infancy but it's growing at such a rate. There are students joining medical school now because they want to study it.'

Now, PHEM is just a normal part of life and is a credible option at medical school, attracting some of the brightest and best physicians. 'PHEM is now seen as a core part of training, no longer the domain of oddballs and enthusiasts,' says Gareth.

ABOVE Air ambulances nationwide have steadily developed into highly regarded, consistent, critical pre-hospital care services. Here a Great Western Air Ambulance Charity (GWAAC) crew returns from a call. *(GWAAC)*

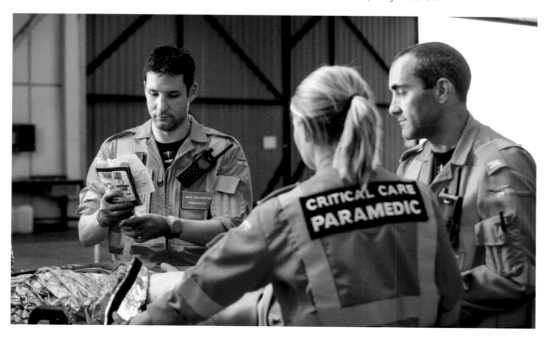

LEFT Training is an ongoing process for all air ambulance crew members. *(GWAAC)*

Origins of air ambulance services in the UK

While air ambulances may now be a familiar sight to most of us, they are in fact a fairly recent development in emergency care. The first air ambulance service was established in Cornwall in 1987 and was the brainchild of aviation consultant Geoff Newman.

An ex-naval helicopter pilot who had served on HMS *Ark Royal*, Geoff had been working for a London-based consultancy, providing advice to various oil companies around the world. In 1986 he found himself in China, working on a bid to supply a helicopter search and rescue capability. During the course of his research,

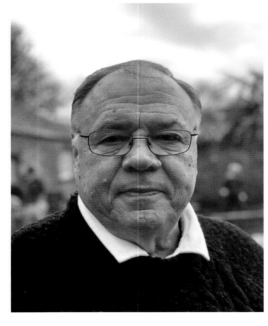

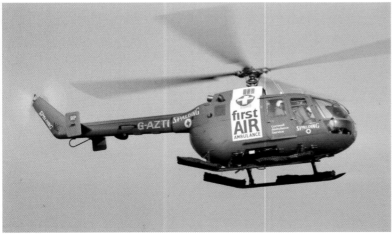

he had been learning about the ways in which public helicopter services worked in other countries and had started looking at how the UK, a nation he describes as being 'full of small helicopters', could more effectively utilise them in similar roles. While Royal Navy helicopters had sometimes been used to transfer difficult spinal injury patients, using military resources for this kind of operation was extremely expensive and impractical compared to using helicopters from the civilian sector. Other countries, such as Germany and France, were using small helicopters to provide supplementary services to their own health services, in the shape of what we now call air ambulances. So why did the UK, a nation rich in aviation history and complete with sophisticated Royal Navy and Royal Air Force Search and Rescue services, not offer the same?

The problem was the way in which the NHS system is organised and funded by central government. Air ambulances do not come cheap. Helicopters are expensive pieces of equipment to start with and the additional cost of fitting them out for emergency medical services is not inconsiderable. Purchasing, equipping and maintaining them, as well as training and recruiting the crew to operate them, would run into millions. The initial outlay to provide a fleet of government-funded air ambulances to service the UK, in addition to the annual running costs, would be prohibitive.

Geoff explored different models of funding for similar services. Commercial sponsorship was a possible solution but, during the course of his research, Geoff learned that the only organisation that could legally transport patients within the 999 system was the ambulance service. Previous attempts to work outside of the ambulance service, using commercial helicopters that used the police command and control system, had not worked out. A charity-funded model seemed to him the most likely route, given the success of similar organisations such as the Royal National Lifeboat Institution (RNLI). A frontline rescue service founded in 1824, the RNLI is one of the UK's richest charities – its income in 2015/16 was almost £184 million.

Geoff and his family lived in Cornwall, a sparsely populated peninsula with only one neighbouring county. The mechanism for funding NHS services was based on population, while the challenging terrain and road system of the county meant that ground ambulance resources were stretched very thin. Having met with the Cornwall ambulance service, who were receptive to the idea of an air ambulance, Geoff contacted Stephen Bond, CEO of Bond Helicopters, who agreed to provide an MBB105 helicopter for three months, at a greatly reduced hourly rate. So Geoff set to work on an operations strategy.

Paramedics as we know them today did not exist at that time, instead ambulance technicians who mastered some of those skills were designated 'extended trained' and it was technicians in this category that joined the team, trained by experienced technician Paul Westaway. Geoff piloted the helicopter and trained the technicians in their co-piloting duties, such as helping to navigate and reading out pre-take-off and pre-landing checklists.

The UK's first air ambulance service began operating on 1 April 1987 (to coincide with the anniversary of the formation of the RAF). Initial funding provided by the local health authority was withdrawn after the first six months and shortly afterwards the First Air Ambulance Service Trust was officially registered as a charity, now known as Cornwall Air Ambulance Trust, to take over running costs of the operation. The Cornwall Air Ambulance became the catalyst for a network of air ambulances across the UK.

The pace of change since then has been rapid and has coincided with the development of the paramedic as a nationally recognised clinician. Since 1987, air ambulances nationwide have steadily developed into highly regarded, consistent, critical pre-hospital care services. HEMS have grown consistently and air ambulance services have continued to evolve through the advancement of both clinical and aviation practice, including new aircraft, the development of night HEMS and greater use of the doctor/paramedic model in critical care teams. There are now 21 HEMS covering the whole of the UK.

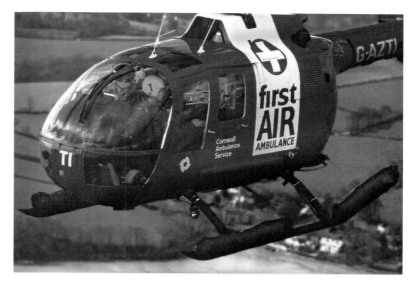

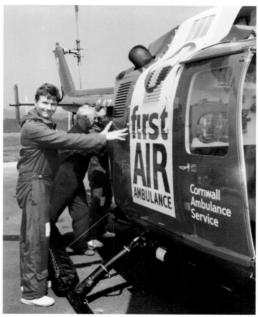

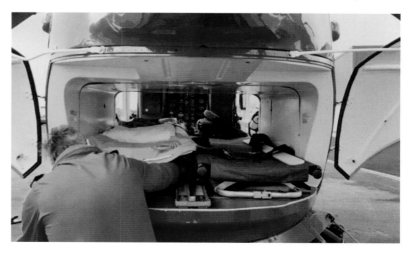

ABOVE 'Tango India' airborne over Cornwall. Note the rearward-facing crew member in the left-hand seat.
(Bond Helicopters)

LEFT Paul Westaway, senior paramedic on the first air ambulance.
(Geoff Newman)

BELOW Patients had to be loaded through the rear of the MBB105 helicopter.
(Geoff Newman)

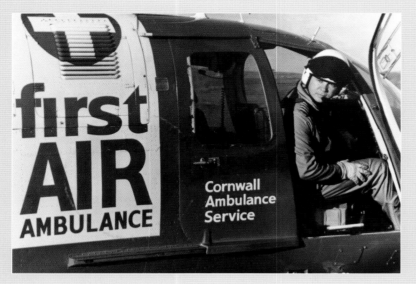

IN THE BEGINNING: CORNWALL'S AIR AMBULANCE

Ex-Royal Navy helicopter pilot and flight instructor Geoff Newman was instrumental in setting up the first UK air ambulance service in Cornwall and was the first person to pilot it.

In its early days, the helicopter operated from a car park outside the Hospital Sterilising Centre at Treliske Hospital (now the Royal Cornwall Hospital). The car park was surrounded by a chain-link fence and the crew worked from a tiny caravan that had previously served as a mobile screening unit. They had a telephone, a fax, a battery cart and tea-making facilities. The nearest A&E hospital in those days was in the centre of Truro and there was a patch of garden nearby that was adequate for the helicopter to land on if the patient needed urgent attention.

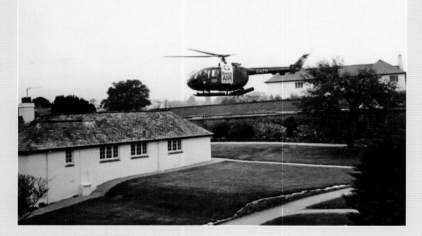

Before the service launched, Geoff had confided in Paul Westaway, a senior paramedic on the air ambulance, that he was apprehensive about dealing with the sight of blood at the scene of an incident. 'Paul recommended a short visit to the morgue,' says Geoff. 'He took me along to observe proceedings and then disappeared, returning four hours later. In the meantime, the mortuary assistants gave me lessons on the conduct of post-mortems and then asked me to assist them with the weighing of organs. It was certainly a unique and valuable experience, although I didn't sleep properly for three days afterwards. But it seemed to do the trick.'

On their first day of operation, a call came

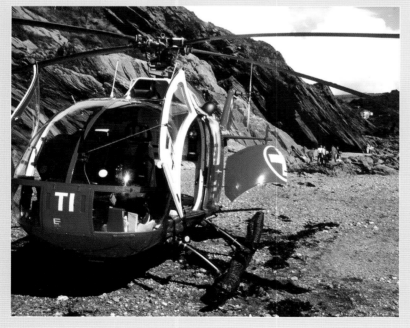

TOP Geoff Newman at the helm of Tango India, the UK's first air ambulance.

CENTRE Truro City Hospital had a patch of garden that functioned as a helipad. The site was so small that it was considered high risk, so rather than expose the crew to departures from it, Geoff would take the aircraft out by himself and rendezvous with the two crew at the helipad at Treliske Hospital. (Paul Westaway)

LEFT Incidents on Cornwall's beaches and coastal paths were attended regularly. (Geoff Newman)

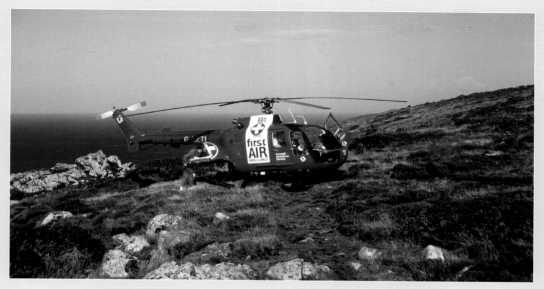

LEFT The Cornish
service became
a catalyst for the
rest of the UK's air
ambulances.
(Geoff Newman)

BELOW The helicopter
operated from a car
park outside the
Hospital Sterilising
Centre at Treliske
Hospital. It was kept in
a parking area, along
with a fuel bowser,
battery pack and
standby ambulance.
The ambulance was
allocated to conduct
transfers to A&E if
the local vehicle was
unavailable. If poor
weather meant no
helicopter service
could be provided,
Control would use the
crew along with this
ambulance for local
calls. *(Geoff Newman)*

in from Porthcurno, where a young woman
had received a spinal injury when rock
climbing. The land ambulance at the scene had
requested assistance – the patient needed to
be transported with the utmost care, due to the
nature of her injury, but was located a long way
from their vehicle, across a sandy beach.

'Once we had delivered her to Treliske
Hospital,' recalls Geoff, 'she looked up at
paramedic Nigel Harris and said: "This is a
wonderful service you have here in Cornwall,
how long have you been running?" Nigel looked
at his watch and replied: "Since about 8.30 this
morning, actually."'

When Geoff left Cornwall Air Ambulance,
he went on to work all over the world as a
pilot, consultant, instructor and manager,
including a ten-year stint as a training
instructor at the AgustaWestland (now
Leonardo Helicopters) training academy in
Italy. He also worked as a search and rescue
pilot in Ireland and spent two years as chief
pilot of London's Air Ambulance.

Now retired and still living in Cornwall, Geoff
has turned his hand to writing and is author
of *The Genesis of the Cornwall Air Ambulance
Service*, his personal account of how the first
UK air ambulance came into being.

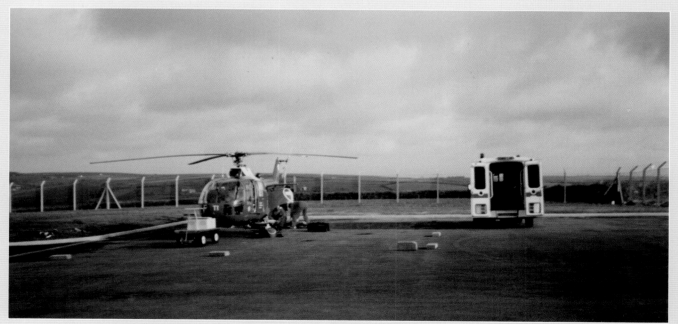

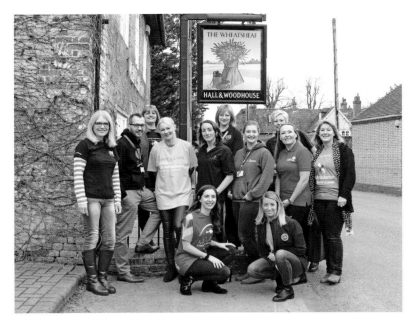

Funding

While they may be tasked via a 999 call and transport NHS clinicians to a patient's side, most air ambulances in the UK are not part of the NHS, receive no direct government funding and no support from the National Lottery, but instead are funded by charitable organisations.

The only exception to this is Scotland which, in addition to a charity-funded air ambulance, is also served by helicopters and fixed-wing aircraft belonging to the Scottish Air Ambulance that are funded entirely from the public purse as part of the wider Scottish ambulance service. The NHS service provided in Scotland differs significantly in that its main role is inter-hospital transfer and retrieval. This is largely driven by the geography of the country, with many patients living in the extremely remote areas of the Highlands and Islands.

Air ambulance services in the UK did not come into being as the result of a central strategy, they rose from a desire within communities to complement and enhance the existing NHS ambulance service provision – and the formation of charities was the only affordable way of achieving this goal without having to make savings elsewhere. Other than the Scottish Air Ambulance, each of the 21 HEMS in the UK is run by a charity and every charity works extremely hard to raise the

necessary funds to support its own aircraft and clinical teams. In 2018, this network of air ambulance charities raised over £180 million across the UK, thanks to a committed band of volunteers, staff and trustees – and, of course, the companies and members of the public who donated their money.

On the face of it, it may seem scandalous that such a vital emergency service has to be run by charities rather than funded by government, but scratch beneath the surface and there are a number of compelling reasons why the charity model is so effective at the moment. Government funding would certainly provide a degree of assurance, but in reality, there would be no consistent or reliable commitment to what the level of funding would actually be in any particular area – the disparity of NHS funding from region to region is in the news all the time.

Air ambulances would probably feature pretty low in terms of priority when it came to ambulance service funding and budget, because they actually care for a very small percentage of the ambulance services' overall cases. Air ambulance services in the UK deal with approximately 70–80 cases per day, which is nothing compared to the ambulance service – in October 2018 alone, for example, the ambulance service received an average of 22,419 calls per day.

Another downside to being government-funded organisations is that they would be subject to the political priorities of others and to prohibitive levels of bureaucracy. When it comes to key issues, such as purchasing expensive helicopters, for example, an air ambulance charity has the flexibility that many government-run organisations do not, meaning it can be more agile and make decisions quickly.

Association of Air Ambulances

With air ambulances playing such a crucial role in saving lives, close co-operation between the different services and related industries is key to ensuring that patient well-being remains top priority when responding to an incident. While each of the services operate well within their own silos, in operational and clinical terms air ambulances must be borderless.

At the heart of each air ambulance charity and its HEMS is the aspiration for clinical and operational excellence, consistency of clinical practice and sound underpinning governance – all focused solely on improving patient care. All of these elements are enshrined in the Association of Air Ambulances' (AAA) Vision Statement: 'The AAA's vision is to improve patient outcomes through the provision of outstanding services to its members.'

The AAA is the trade body representing all organisations that form part of the UK air ambulance service. While it primarily represents

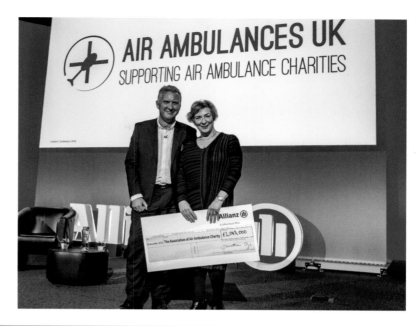

RIGHT Air Ambulances UK (formerly the Association of Air Ambulances Charity) filters national donations that local air ambulances cannot access.

ALL-PARTY PARLIAMENTARY GROUP FOR AIR AMBULANCES

A key function of the AAA is to raise the quality of care and effectiveness of air ambulances for patients through engagement with political leaders and policy makers and the Association is the secretariat for the All-Party Parliamentary Group for Air Ambulances (APPGAA).

All-Party Parliamentary Groups are informal, cross-party groups formed by MPs and members of the House of Lords who share a common interest in a particular policy area, region or country. When AAA became an incorporated body in 2012, it set up the APPGAA to lobby with members of the Commons and Lords on key issues that impact the air ambulance community. This included operational issues, such as providing helipads at hospitals; clinical issues, like flight time limitations for pilots and clinicians; and charity issues, such as the cap on lottery funding.

Because charities can't lobby and must stay apolitical, the APPGAA gave the AAA the opportunity to lobby for the air ambulance sector. It also allowed the Association to pursue and gain access to the banking fines and LIBOR funds that were made available by then-Chancellor of the Exchequer George Osborne.

In 2013, the AAA was instructed by the Home Secretary to obtain bids from air ambulances to receive a share of the LIBOR funds. The money had to go towards capital expenditure, not just operational costs, so projects such as a base build or rebuild, a training centre or a new aircraft. The Treasury awarded £5 million to the AAA and the Association then set up a service charity (the Air Ambulance Association Charity) in order to disperse the funds. Having its foot in Westminster's door with the APPGAA meant the AAA could ensure that air ambulances weren't missed off the services charity list when the Chancellor announced that was where the funds were directed.

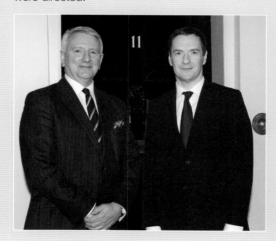

LEFT In 2015, then-Chancellor of the Exchequer George Osborne (pictured here with DSAA Chief Executive Bill Sivewright) awarded £250,000 from the LIBOR fines fund to DSAA, which enabled it to upgrade its operational facilities.

NATIONAL AIR AMBULANCE WEEK

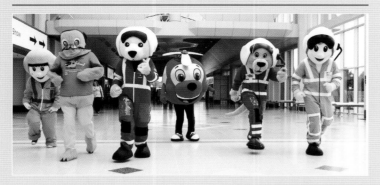

ABOVE Air ambulance mascots come out to support National Air Ambulance Week, which is held annually to raise awareness, and provide a boost to fundraising efforts.

One of the AAA's tasks is to raise exposure of the sector in the public eye. The main way in which this is achieved is through National Air Ambulance Week (NAAW), which takes place during the second week of September each year. The initiative celebrates the work of local air ambulance charities across the UK and gives them a national platform from which to promote their efforts, raise money and increase awareness among the general public.

Many of the charities organise fundraising and awareness-raising events in which celebrities, businesses and members of the public show their support by getting involved.

The first NAAW was held in 2012 and the AAA described it as a significant success for air ambulance charities, raising awareness and providing a welcome boost to fundraising efforts. Both local and national media picked up on the event, which was supported by then-patron Sir David Jason, paving the way for the annual event to grow in both size and popularity.

In 2018, the air ambulance charities collectively raised over £180 million, operated 36 helicopters and flew on average 20,500 missions each year, supported by a volunteer network of more than 5,000 people.

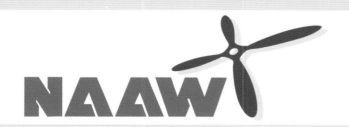

those in the front line who treat patients, it also spans the entire network; the charitable trusts, the operators, ambulance services and associated trades. When it comes to clinical care, the needs of the patient are always the priority, so the AAA does not advocate a specific model of care, but instead recognises the need for services that are tailored to meet the demands of the different local care environments.

Together with a handful of other ambulance service chief executives, David Philpott of Kent, Surrey and Sussex Air Ambulance helped establish the Association of Air Ambulance Charities (as it was then known) in 2006. David drafted the original constitution and was appointed after a unanimous vote by charity CEOs to become the founding chairman, spending three years in the post.

The AAA had a simple vision and a simple remit. It would be a low-subscription, mutual support body for air ambulance charity CEOs, advocating dialogue and information sharing. It would also co-ordinate national fundraising initiatives and provide a single industry voice for government and the helicopter industry on matters of mutual concern.

Today, the Association has expanded and now endeavours to build on existing relationships between all parties to develop a continually improving emergency response network, as well as working with its members to promote best practice at all times. It is funded by subscriptions from the air ambulance services, as well as from associate members who are suppliers to the sector – aircraft manufacturers and operators, lottery providers and so on.

It also acts in an advisory capacity in a number of ways. Sometimes, people who have died leave legacies to 'the air ambulance' but are not specific about which one, or they leave legacies to a particular organisation – 'West Midlands Air Ambulance', for example – when there is no service by that name. As the umbrella organisation for all air ambulance services in the UK, the AAA can help advise solicitors on where these legacies should go.

The organisation also provides assistance to other countries that are setting up air ambulance services. Very little advisory material existed in this sector, so a few years ago the AAA

AIR AMBULANCE AWARDS

Held each year, the Air Ambulance Awards of Excellence are an opportunity to recognise the work of those in the air ambulance sector, from the experienced personnel who task the air ambulance to the skilled pilots, the highly trained clinicians, the hard-working charity staff and the committed fundraising teams who help to keep their respective services flying. The awards are open to any individual or team within the air ambulance community in the UK, and recognise exceptional people in the following categories:

- Outstanding Young Person Award
- Charity Staff Member of the Year
- Air Ambulance Paramedic of the Year
- Air Ambulance Doctor of the Year
- Air Ambulance Pilot of the Year
- Air Ambulance Campaign of the Year
- Charity Volunteer of the Year
- Air Ambulance Innovation Award
- Special Incident Award

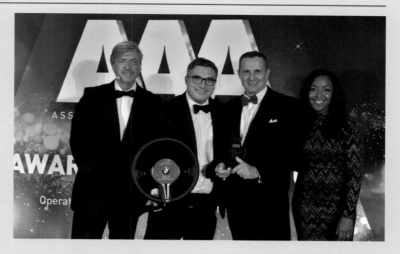

ABOVE AAA's Air Ambulance Paramedic of the Year 2018 was awarded to Mark Williams of Dorset and Somerset Air Ambulance. Pictured here with TV presenter Richard Madeley; Chris Leamonth, MD of BMW Park Lane, sponsor of the award; and Angellica Bell, presenter.

- Air Operations Support Staff Member of the Year
- Lifetime Achievement Award.

published a *Framework for a High Performing Ambulance Service*, which was created to give the layperson an insight into how the sector works. Using this same framework, AAA is now helping countries such as Costa Rica, South Korea and Indonesia. These countries are keen to develop air ambulance services in a pre-hospital care environment but don't always know where to start, how to staff a service or how to obtain the right level of clinical knowledge. Funding models vary throughout the world, so advice is also available on how to fund a fledgling service; there are private models, state-funded models and insurance models, with only the UK, Norway and New Zealand currently using the charitable model.

Essentially, the AAA provides the bridge between air ambulance charities, ambulance services and the wider supply chain, enabling clinical best practice to be shared, helping to co-ordinate fundraising and improving efficiency. This process of continual improvement through collaboration is key to the ongoing success of air ambulance services in the UK.

Air ambulances in the UK

While each of the 21 air ambulance services covers a specific geographical area, in operational and clinical terms the air ambulance service is borderless. If, for example, an incident arises in Cornwall but the Cornwall Air Ambulance Trust helicopters are unavailable, the Devon Air Ambulance Trust would be tasked by South Western Ambulance Service Foundation Trust (SWASFT) instead. When major incidents occur, a number of different air ambulance services may be tasked: some to convey more clinicians to the site of the incident because of the pre-hospital care they can provide, some to transfer patients to the nearest appropriate hospital.

Hospitals with landing sites

Many hospitals don't need to have a dedicated helicopter landing site or helipad, as they will never be the first receiver for the most urgent cases. But for major trauma centres (MTCs) and larger regional hospitals, the ability to

continued on page 32

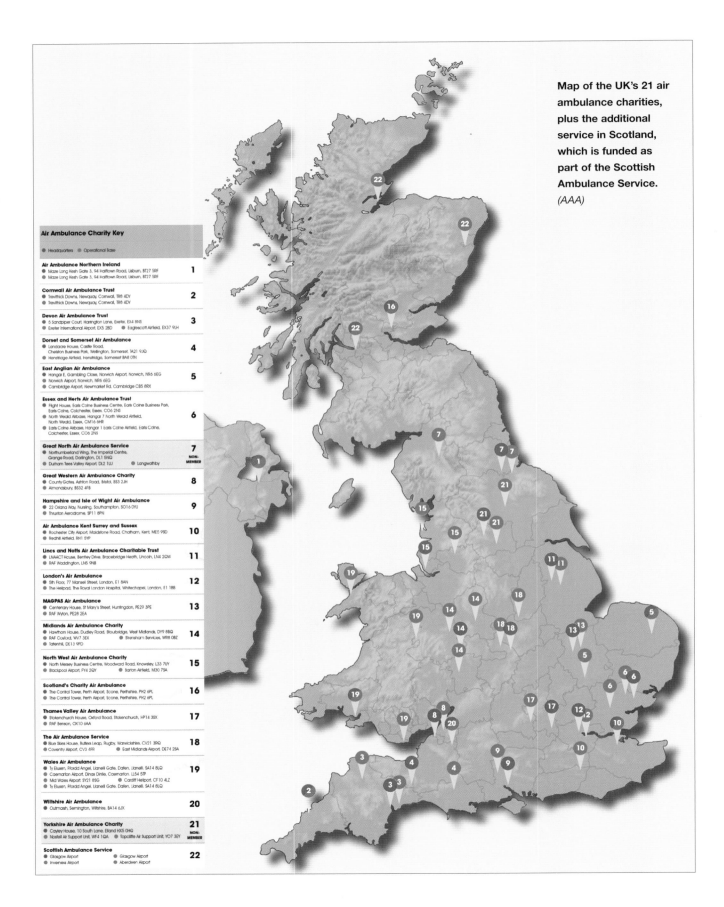

Map of the UK's 21 air ambulance charities, plus the additional service in Scotland, which is funded as part of the Scottish Ambulance Service.
(AAA)

Major Trauma Centres

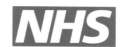

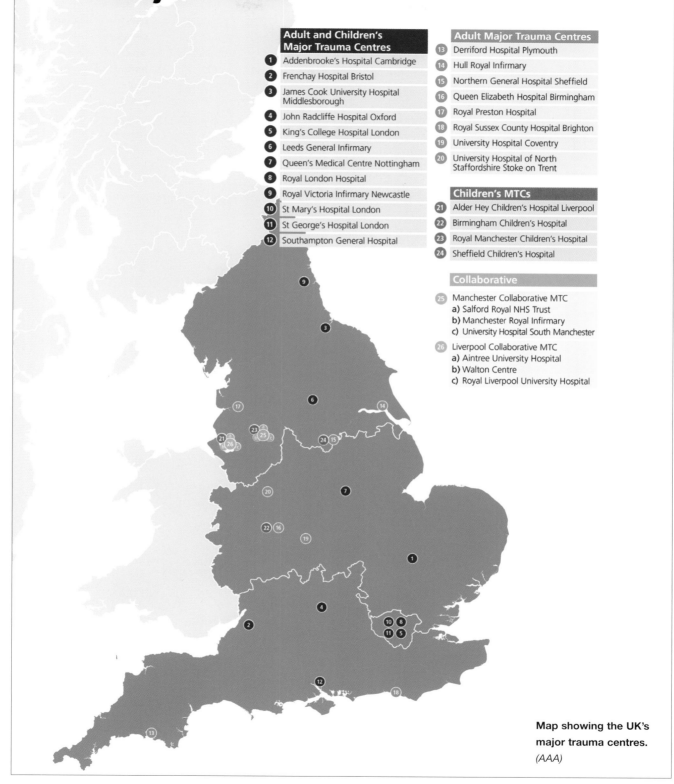

Adult and Children's Major Trauma Centres

1. Addenbrooke's Hospital Cambridge
2. Frenchay Hospital Bristol
3. James Cook University Hospital Middlesborough
4. John Radcliffe Hospital Oxford
5. King's College Hospital London
6. Leeds General Infirmary
7. Queen's Medical Centre Nottingham
8. Royal London Hospital
9. Royal Victoria Infirmary Newcastle
10. St Mary's Hospital London
11. St George's Hospital London
12. Southampton General Hospital

Adult Major Trauma Centres

13. Derriford Hospital Plymouth
14. Hull Royal Infirmary
15. Northern General Hospital Sheffield
16. Queen Elizabeth Hospital Birmingham
17. Royal Preston Hospital
18. Royal Sussex County Hospital Brighton
19. University Hospital Coventry
20. University Hospital of North Staffordshire Stoke on Trent

Children's MTCs

21. Alder Hey Children's Hospital Liverpool
22. Birmingham Children's Hospital
23. Royal Manchester Children's Hospital
24. Sheffield Children's Hospital

Collaborative

25. Manchester Collaborative MTC
   a) Salford Royal NHS Trust
   b) Manchester Royal Infirmary
   c) University Hospital South Manchester
26. Liverpool Collaborative MTC
   a) Aintree University Hospital
   b) Walton Centre
   c) Royal Liverpool University Hospital

Map showing the UK's major trauma centres.
(AAA)

Air ambulances are often called out to road traffic accidents and those that involve motorcyclists often have an unhappy outcome. When a motorcyclist has a collision, they have no roll cage, no airbag and no metal chassis to protect them. It doesn't matter how quickly help arrives, how much blood the clinical team is carrying or what level of skills the attending clinicians have, the forces of a collision are often simply too great for the biker to survive. A high proportion of motorcyclists travelling at speed will die at the scene of an incident.

Ian Mew is an intensive care consultant at Dorset County Hospital and its former director of major trauma, where he was responsible for the care of those who had been involved in serious accidents. He also flies with Dorset and Somerset Air Ambulance (DSAA).

It was clear to Ian, who has been a keen motorcyclist since the age of 16, that it was not enough to simply pick up the pieces at the roadside. Instead, focusing on injury prevention by reaching motorcyclists before they have

a crash would be a far more effective way to prevent deaths.

Ian is a former chief medical officer for the Dorset Police and, together with a colleague, PC Chris Smith from Dorset Police BikeSafe, they came up with the DocBike initiative, which aims to reduce the number of motorcycle deaths through engagement, injury prevention, education and roadside critical care.

'Putting a non-police person on a high-profile bike allows them to engage more effectively with motorcyclists, who are often less keen to deal with authority figures like the police,' explains Ian. 'An air ambulance doctor on a high-profile motorbike is a real draw. We can attend large biker events and people will come and have a chat with us, so it works well as an engagement tool.' Using an ex-police bike, rebadged as DocBike, Ian is also able to deliver critical care at the roadside.

The DocBike project delivers life-saving skills to riders through free BikerDown courses, which are held at events across the UK. The three-module course designed by Kent Fire &

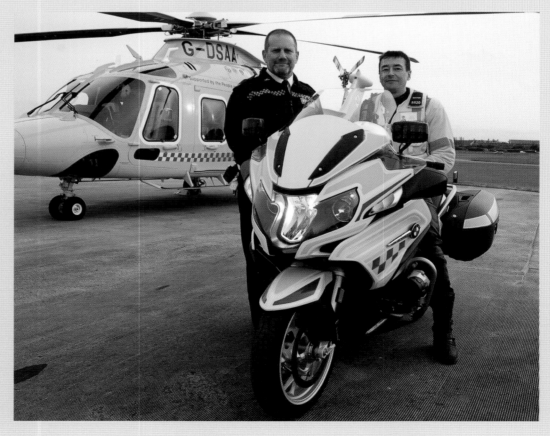

RIGHT Dr Ian Mew and PC Chris Smith, founders of the DocBike initiative, which aims to reduce the number of motorcyclist deaths in the UK.

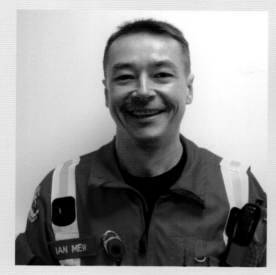

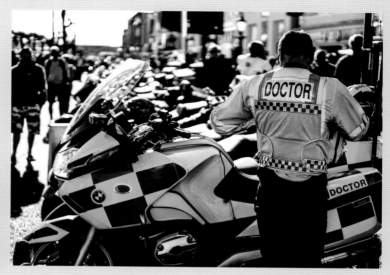

Rescue Service teaches riders about scene safety and how to keep someone alive, as well as how to avoid being in a collision themselves. The DocBike uses this last module to signpost riders to further courses that will specifically improve their awareness of why motorcycle collisions occur and help them to avoid being in a collision themselves.

DocBike is a national charity, which has forged links with the National Police Chiefs Council, the National Fire Chiefs Council and the Association of Ambulance Chief Executives, all of whom have given their backing. 'It's important to get this top-level collaboration in order to push the programme out nationally,' says Ian.

DSAA has also embraced the concept of injury prevention and is helping to spread the message. Another DSAA doctor, Rob Török, works with the Safe Drive Stay Alive project, while Medical Lead Phil Hyde has chaired the injury prevention arm of the Trauma Care Conference.

'We want to change the culture of how motorcyclists are riding,' says Ian. 'Not saying "slow down", but instead raising awareness of what is most likely to kill them. If you approach a junction too quickly, for example, and a car does pull out in front of you, you need to make sure you have enough time to avoid the collision. If riders can do that instinctively because they understand and are aware of the dangers, they are more likely to react in the right way.'

Awareness of invisibility is also a key factor. Ian's analogy is to imagine a dart being thrown at your face: you either won't see it coming or, if you do, you won't perceive its speed in time for you to catch it. If motorcyclists understand that is how they appear to drivers waiting to pull out at a junction, particularly when riding at speed, they can modify their behaviour accordingly.

Research undertaken by the Trauma Audit and Research Network and Dorset Police Traffic Department looked at all the motorcycle injuries and deaths in Dorset over a two-year period. It concluded that 80% of motorcyclists would not have been in the collision that resulted in their death or critical injury, had they been riding safely for the circumstances.

'We specifically don't tell motorcyclists to stick to the speed limit because we know they won't,' says Ian. 'It's pointless and they will just disengage. Instead we highlight the areas where using excessive speed will put them at real risk of being killed because they won't have time to react.'

Now the infrastructure is in place, DocBike can be scaled up, so Ian is in talks with a number of other air ambulance services. As the initiative grows, more air ambulance clinicians will be needed across the country to take DocBikes to events, draw the audience in and then encourage them to take BikerDown courses.

Although the charity is in its infancy when it comes to securing funding, it has engaged a PhD student from Bournemouth University for three years to carry out in-depth research. 'There's no point having more bikes out there yet if we don't know if what we are doing is effective,' says Ian. 'Research is key to everything we do.' Once the evidence is in place, it will be easier to bring others on board to help deliver an effective injury prevention strategy.

ABOVE LEFT Ian Mew, former chief medical officer for the Dorset Police, is an intensive care consultant with Dorset County Hospital and also flies with DSAA.

ABOVE Doctors on high-profile bikes are able to engage with bikers on the subject of safety.

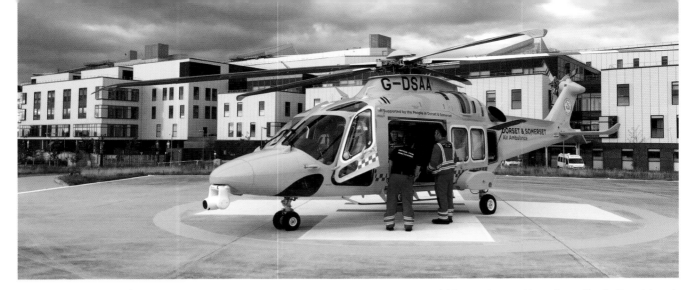

ABOVE **The Dorset and Somerset Air Ambulance frequently lands at Southmead Hospital in Bristol.**

BELOW **Helipads are as critical to hospitals as land ambulance access.**
(Leonardo Helicopters)

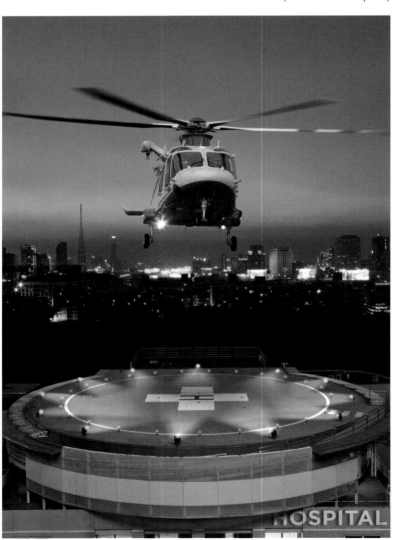

quickly receive and transfer critically ill or injured patients from the air ambulance and into the hospital is vital.

The AAA has produced a map of the hospitals and MTCs that have some form of accessibility for an air ambulance, whether it is a state-of-the-art helipad or a secondary landing site such as a patch of nearby tarmac or grass. A report by the AAA's operational subcommittee detailed the provision of hospital landing sites (HLS) in the UK and outlined a number of criteria to define the quality of an HLS:

- Is the HLS located on the hospital grounds or offsite?
- What is the proximity of the HLS to the emergency department and will staff be able to take the patient directly to the emergency department or is there the requirement for the patient to be offloaded from the air ambulance into a land ambulance and then driven to the emergency department by road?
- Is the surface of the HLS grass, meaning that in times of adverse weather use of the HLS may increase risk to staff, or even result in the HLS being closed, with the hospital losing its ability to receive patients?
- Is the HLS staffed by security or clinical staff to ensure the safe operation during landing and take-off and transfer of patients into the hospital?
- Is the HLS of a suitable size and lit in accordance with regulations to enable air ambulances to land with patients during the hours of darkness?
- Is the route from the HLS suitably screened and covered to maintain patient dignity and

the safety of staff if there is adverse weather during the transfer from the air ambulance to the emergency department?

Helipads should be considered as critical to hospitals as land ambulance access, but even when it is possible to install one, it is a costly exercise. The County Air Ambulance Trust, a charity established in the early 1990s, originally to support the West Midlands ambulance service, launched the HELP Appeal in 2009. Its aim is to raise funds in order to provide grants to help fund helipads at major hospitals and MTCs around the UK. In most cases, the HELP Appeal funds 100% of the costs for each helipad, but where there is a shortfall, the hospitals contribute the remaining amount needed. The very first helipad funded by the HELP Appeal was at the Robert Jones and Agnes Hunt Orthopaedic Hospital in Oswestry, a leading orthopaedic centre of excellence. To date, the appeal has funded 25 new and upgraded helipads, with another 44 in the pipeline.

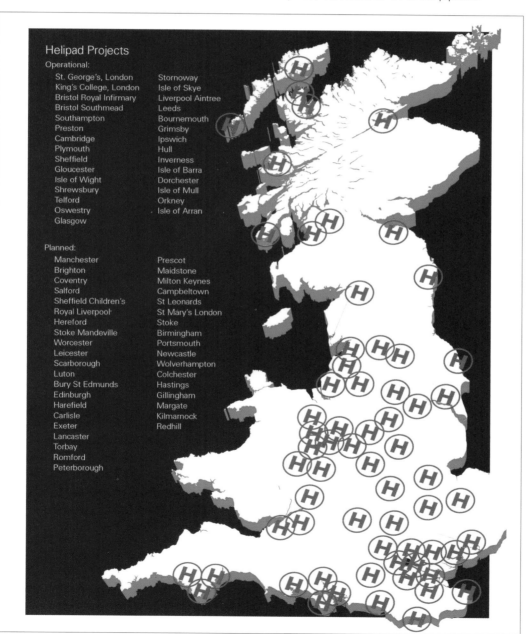

Helipad Projects

Operational:

St. George's, London	Stornoway
King's College, London	Isle of Skye
Bristol Royal Infirmary	Liverpool Aintree
Bristol Southmead	Leeds
Southampton	Bournemouth
Preston	Grimsby
Cambridge	Ipswich
Plymouth	Hull
Sheffield	Inverness
Gloucester	Isle of Barra
Isle of Wight	Dorchester
Shrewsbury	Isle of Mull
Telford	Orkney
Oswestry	Isle of Arran
Glasgow	

Planned:

Manchester	Prescot
Brighton	Maidstone
Coventry	Milton Keynes
Salford	Campbeltown
Sheffield Children's	St Leonards
Royal Liverpool	St Mary's London
Hereford	Stoke
Stoke Mandeville	Birmingham
Worcester	Portsmouth
Leicester	Newcastle
Scarborough	Wolverhampton
Luton	Colchester
Bury St Edmunds	Hastings
Edinburgh	Gillingham
Harefield	Margate
Carlisle	Kilmarnock
Exeter	Redhill
Lancaster	
Torbay	
Romford	
Peterborough	

LEFT Map showing the completed and planned helipad projects funded by the HELP Appeal.
(HELP Appeal)

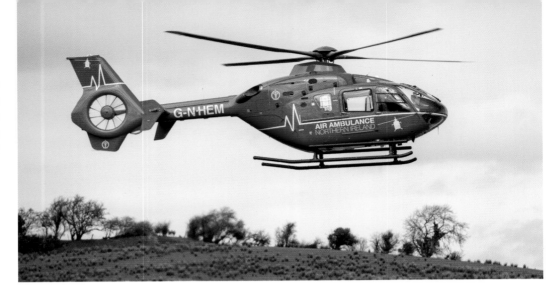

Regional air ambulance services

Air Ambulance Northern Ireland (AANI)

AANI works in partnership with the Northern Ireland ambulance service to provide HEMS for the region. It has one operational helicopter and one back-up helicopter, as well as a rapid response vehicle. AANI's EC135 helicopter can get anywhere in the province in approximately 25–30 minutes and operates for 12 hours a day, 365 days a year. Launched in July 2017, AANI has a landing base at the former Maze prison site in Lisburn, County Antrim and a back-up base at St Angelo, outside Enniskillen.

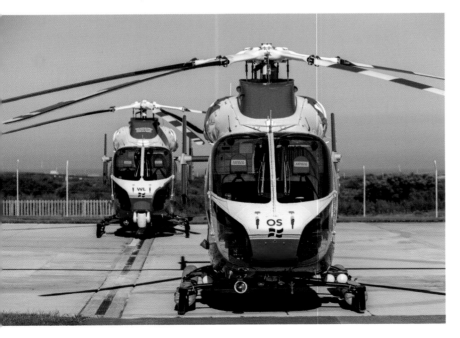

Cornwall Air Ambulance Trust (CAAT)

In a county that contains isolated beaches, remote rural settlements and challenging road networks, Cornwall Air Ambulance is a lifeline to the half a million people who live there, as well as its millions of visitors. Launched in 1987, Cornwall Air Ambulance was the first air ambulance in the UK, operating throughout Cornwall and the Isles of Scilly. Since the service began it has completed more than 28,000 missions, with a paramedic aircrew providing pre-hospital care at the scene of the incident and flying patients to specialist hospital units in Cornwall, Devon, Bristol and even Swansea. CAAT currently operates two MD 902 Explorers and relies on its supporters for its running costs of £3.5 million a year. In 2018, the charity launched a £2.5m appeal to bring a new AW169 air ambulance to Cornwall and the Isles of Scilly.

Devon Air Ambulance Trust (DAAT)

After her son, Ceri, was knocked from his bike and killed in 1986, Devon resident Ann Thomas was told that his chances of survival would have been improved if he had received treatment earlier. Ann then launched the Ceri Thomas Appeal to raise funds to provide Devon with an air ambulance. She succeeded and on 27 August 1992, Devon Air Ambulance flew its first mission. Initially flying five days a week, the service was extended to seven days a week in 1997. The county of Devon spans a huge geographical area, with two coastlines, hundreds of remote villages and acres of

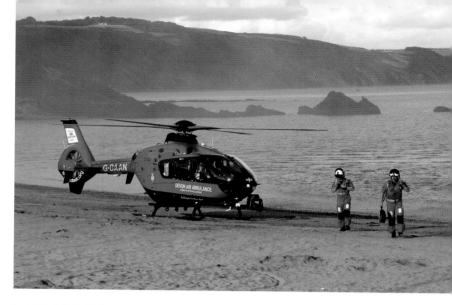

RIGHT One of Devon Air Ambulance Trust's two
EC135s in action. *(DAAT)*

rural wilderness, which is covered by the two
Eurocopter EC135s that the charity owns.

Dorset and Somerset Air Ambulance (DSAA)

Launched in 2000, DSAA operates its AW169
helicopter from Henstridge Airfield in Somerset,
close to the Dorset border. In 2017 it introduced
night HEMS, enabling the service to run for 19
hours a day, every day of the year. The next
chapter looks at the service's operation in detail.

East Anglian Air Ambulance (EAAA)

EAAA launched in 2000 as a one-day-a-week
service with a helicopter and a crew consisting
of one pilot and one paramedic. By January
2019, EAAA, which covers the four counties
of Norfolk, Suffolk, Cambridgeshire and
Bedfordshire, had flown its 25,000th mission
with a crew now consisting of two pilots, a
doctor and a critical care paramedic.

The charity operates two H145 helicopters,
one located at Norwich Airport and the other
at Cambridge Airport, with two rapid response
vehicles also supporting the operation. The
crew treat patients who have suffered life-
threatening accidents or medical emergencies

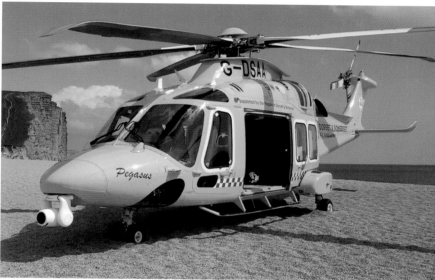

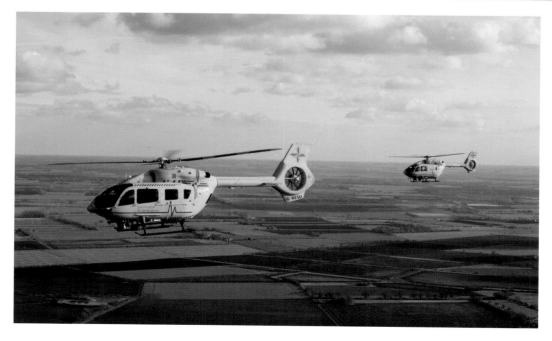

ABOVE Dorset
and Somerset Air
Ambulance upgraded
its aircraft to an
AW169 in 2017.
(Phil Merritt)

LEFT East Anglian
Air Ambulance covers
four counties with its
two H145 helicopters.
(EAAA)

continued on page ??

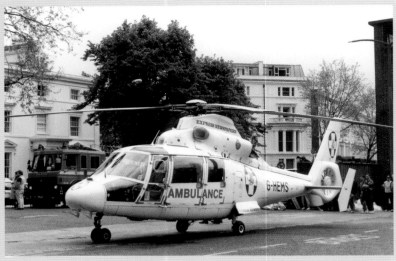

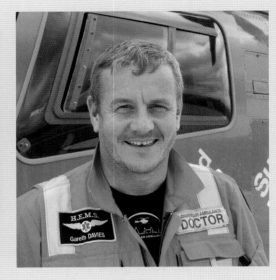

LONDON'S AIR AMBULANCE

London's Air Ambulance is unique in a number of ways. While most of the UK's air ambulances serve a mixture of urban and rural populations, London's Air Ambulance works almost exclusively within the confines of the M25. It covers around 600 square miles and serves a population that swells to around 10 million during the day, including all those who commute in to the capital. This workload and nature of the missions it carries out is different to almost any air ambulance worldwide.

Based at the Royal London Hospital in Whitechapel, London's Air Ambulance launched in January 1989 as HEMS London and was set up as a joint initiative between the hospital, the *Daily Express* newspaper and the NHS. Its first mission was to collect some donor organs for transplantation from Scotland, and it flew from its base (which was then at Biggin Hill Airfield) with just a pilot and paramedic on board. Now the service operates two helicopters and five rapid response vehicles, and during the 30 years it has been flying its clinical team has treated around 40,000 patients, attending some 2,000 missions every year.

Its two MD 902 Explorer helicopters fly only during daylight hours, with an average flight time of six minutes, and only need an area of around

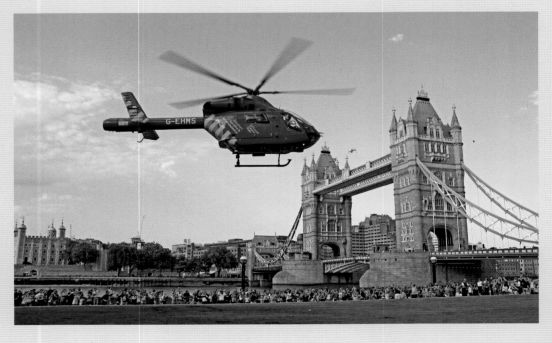

80 square feet (the size of a tennis court) to land. The doctor-paramedic crew only attends trauma, such as road traffic collisions (which, unlike the rest of the country, mainly involve cyclists or pedestrians), penetrating trauma (shootings and stabbings) and falls from height. About once a week the team also attends someone under a train on the underground, Dockland Light Railway or overground, another situation unique to London and one that presents extra challenges for the entire crew.

In most cases, the clinical team is flown to the patient to treat them at the scene, before accompanying them in a land ambulance to the appropriate major trauma centre. Only around one quarter of patients are airlifted to hospital. Trauma cases provide a heavy workload and the crew can attend to five or six patients every shift.

As well as a huge population, London also has some of the most crowded airspace in the world and London's Air Ambulance has the unique privilege of being prioritised over all other air traffic when on an emergency call. Landings often happen on playing fields, parks, school playgrounds and tennis courts and the pilots are working in a very complex environment. For this reason, the service operates a two-pilot model and medical crew members are not required to directly assist with aviation duties.

The MD 902 Explorer was selected for a number of reasons, including its overall size, its excellent all-round visibility from the cockpit and its relatively small disc size in terms of the main rotors. It has no tail rotors and a very high main rotor clearance, which is essential in an environment where members of the public are likely to be present. The Explorer was also chosen because of its skids, as they require less maintenance. The previous aircraft had wheels, but the extreme wear and tear that occurred from having to put them up and down numerous times a day meant that they were not suitable in the long term.

Clinical operation

London's Air Ambulance has pioneered a number of techniques in pre-hospital care. It was the first air ambulance service to provide pre-hospital anaesthesia, perform pre-hospital resuscitative thoracotomy, carry blood and perform pre-hospital resuscitative endovascular balloon occlusion of the aorta (known as REBOA).

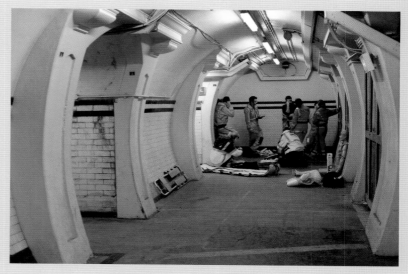

The driving force behind much of this work is Medical Director Gareth Davies. An emergency physician by training, Gareth joined the service in 1993 as a registrar and was the first-ever NHS appointment in pre-hospital care back in 1996. His role over the past 25 years has been about developing the service and its clinical governance framework, recruiting and training the doctors and paramedics and quality assuring the care that the service delivers.

ABOVE Attending to patients who have fallen under a train on the underground is a situation unique to London and one that presents extra challenges for the crew. *(London's Air Ambulance)*

BELOW The MD 902 Explorer has no tail rotors (NOTAR) and a very high main rotor clearance – vital in an environment where members of the public are often present. *(Matthew Bell)*

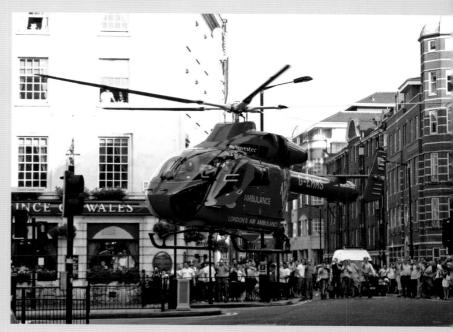

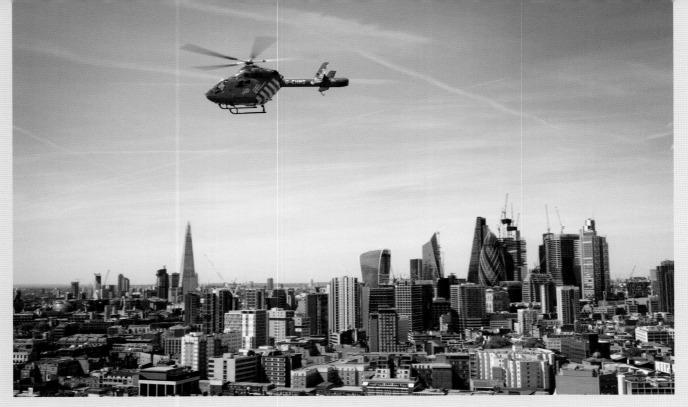

The clinical operation at London's Air Ambulance differs from most other services in several ways. The doctors are paid for by the NHS (Bart's Health NHS Trust) and the paramedics by the London Ambulance Service, while the charity pays for the helicopter, cars, pilots, engineering, fuel and other operating costs.

Competition to join the team is fierce and the service is more interested in the type of people it appoints than in their specific experience – in Gareth's words: 'People with huge amounts of humility matched by huge amounts of ability.' Around half of the doctors are emergency physicians by background, just under half are anaesthetists and intensivists, and the remainder are from a whole range of disciplines, including neurosurgery, trauma surgery and orthopaedics.

Registrars and paramedics are only in post for six and nine months respectively before being replaced. Gareth and his team have created a model where doctors are brought in, trained up and then sent back out into the wider NHS to spread their skillsets – ostensibly to help create the specialty of pre-hospital emergency medicine.

The training programme is very structured and intense. There is an initial period of mentoring for a month, with the trainee crewed alongside someone who is already signed off to fly solo in the air ambulance. During that month they will learn policy and procedures, as well as how to handle the equipment. This is followed by a formal sign-off procedure, with mentors running through scenarios and trainees attending live missions before being finally assessed by one of the consultants.

This presents quite a high training burden, as every six months doctors have to be educated and trained and they soon go elsewhere. But this is all part of the plan to propagate the message about pre-hospital care. 'Many of our staff went to other UK services but many also went to other countries,' says Gareth. Sydney HEMS, for example, is now led by a team of doctors who had training in London and took many of their practices down under.

'We are very privileged and fortunate to attract some of the best doctors from across the world, including Iceland, Norway, Finland, Germany, Denmark, Canada, Australia and New Zealand,' he continues. 'They have usually been very senior doctors who have come specifically for the sort of training we can give them, as well as exposure to the sort of clinical governance that we have, then taken that away and embedded a similar philosophy and procedures wherever they end up.'

Gareth once flew with an air ambulance in Tromso in Norway and discovered one of his checklists for anaesthesia, translated into Norwegian, in a pack in the cabin. 'It's enormously rewarding to know some of our procedures are embedded in the Arctic Circle, as well as on the other side of the world in Australia and New Zealand,' he says.

Wanting to also propagate the understanding of pre-hospital medicine into the London Ambulance Service, London's Air Ambulance followed the same model with its paramedics, training literally hundreds of paramedics who have gone on to become leaders in their own right, both in the capital and throughout the country.

While none of this would have been possible without the funding provided by the charity, for Gareth this presents an ideological dilemma. 'There's a part of me that has always hoped that our interaction with the third sector one day won't be necessary,' he says. From a clinician's perspective, he feels that pre-hospital care will only really be embedded as a core discipline when it's fully funded by the NHS – despite most of the public already believing it is. However, in the current climate, where there is a huge amount of competition for the NHS pound, he acknowledges that the charity model is still very necessary.

Gareth also believes his team is uniquely placed to deliver pioneering work. 'Because we are based at a hospital, it does allow this clinical innovation to happen at a fast rate, while it is slightly harder if you are based at an airfield and not working within a large clinical institution,' he says. 'You need a big NHS organisation with all of the processes that exist in them to temper, moderate, hone and finesse the procedures. It is harder to do that as a charitable provider. Living and breathing in a massive institution like Bart's Health is one of the things that has allowed us to create some of these interventions.'

The team at London's Air Ambulance feel a burden on themselves to share what they have and how they learn. 'One thing about being in a big, urban environment is that we get to see very sick patients, five or six times a day, who have been stabbed, shot or run over,' explains Gareth. 'In research terms, we don't want that work and that experience to be wasted. We are on a real learning curve and we need to keep sharing our knowledge.'

and transfer them to the most appropriate hospital for their needs. The charity is currently featured in the More4 documentary series *Emergency Helicopter Medics*.

Essex & Herts Air Ambulance Trust (EHAAT)

Established in 1997, Essex Air Ambulance launched its first helicopter in 1998. In 2007, the Essex Air Ambulance Charity became the Essex & Herts Air Ambulance Trust (EHAAT) and the Herts Air Ambulance became operational in November 2008. In March 2016, EHAAT signed a contract with aircraft operator Specialist Aviation Services (SAS) to secure the purchase and operation of an AW169 (based at North Weald) and signed a ten-year contract with SAS to lease an MD 902 Explorer (based at Earls Colne). In addition to two air ambulances, EHAAT has four rapid response vehicles (RRVs) which operate after sunset and when the aircraft are grounded due to bad weather or unplanned maintenance.

In 2018, EHAAT's helicopters and RRVs were dispatched on 2,241 occasions, 83% of these to incidents in Essex and Hertfordshire. The remainder were to attend patients in neighbouring counties of Suffolk, Bedfordshire, Cambridgeshire, Norfolk, Greater London and Kent.

BELOW Essex & Herts Air Ambulance Trust uses an AW169 and an MD 902 Explorer, as well as four Rapid Response Vehicles. *(EHAAT)*

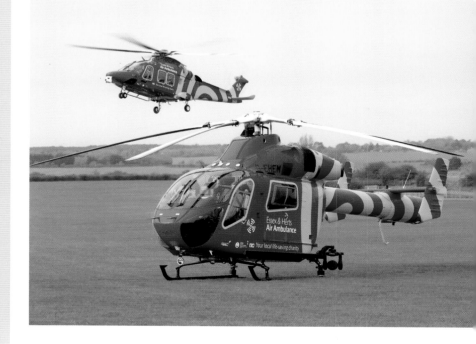

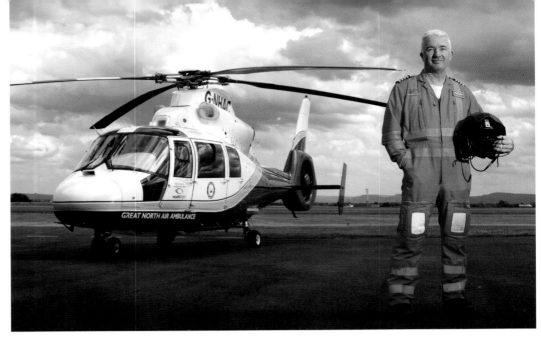

Great North Air Ambulance Service (GNAAS)

The charity's origins can be traced back to 1991, when the Great North Air Ambulance Service Appeal was launched. Four years of hard work (and the generosity of the Barbour Family Trust) saw enough money raised to purchase a helicopter and provide the North East of England's first air ambulance service. Today, with staffed bases at Langwathby and Durham Tees Valley Airport and a forward operating base at Newcastle International Airport, GNAAS's three Eurocopter Dauphin AS365 N2 aircraft cover an area of some 8,000 square miles. The charity owns all three aircraft and they are the only helicopters of their type to be used by a UK air ambulance service.

Great Western Air Ambulance Charity (GWAAC)

One of the busiest air ambulance services in the UK, the GWAAC's EC135 helicopter covers emergencies across Bristol, Bath and North East Somerset, Gloucestershire, North Somerset, South Gloucestershire and surrounding areas. Its crew includes specialist paramedics in critical care and critical care doctors, and it operates from two critical care cars as well as the helicopter, bringing the skills and expertise of an emergency department to the scene of an incident.

On average, GWAAC is called to five incidents every day and its critical care team attended 1,887 jobs in 2018. It is also the youngest service in the UK, having started up in 2008. In 2018, the charity managed to raise £1.25m in order to purchase its airbase in Almondsbury.

Hampshire and Isle of Wight Air Ambulance (HIOWAA)

Operating an Airbus H135 helicopter from its airbase in Thruxton, near Andover, HIOWAA began flying in 2007. The air ambulance, which has been specially equipped and optimised for night operations since 2015, operates alongside a Critical Care Team Vehicle (CCTV). The CCTV is crewed by a team of HIOWAA doctors and paramedics and has parallel capability to the air ambulance. The vehicle, a specially converted Volvo XC90, operates seven days a week, during the day, providing the same enhanced care as that delivered by the air ambulance, but now able to get to the more difficult-to-reach

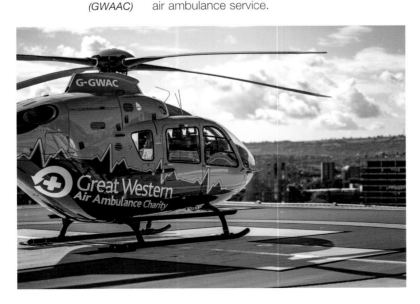

urban areas. On average, HIOWAA attends six missions per day, many of them life-saving. The charity's patron is Lady Montagu, wife of Baron Montagu of Beaulieu, whose estate is home to the National Motor Museum.

Kent, Surrey and Sussex Air Ambulance Trust (KSSAAT)

Having observed the launch of Cornwall and London's air ambulances, KSSAAT founder Kate Chivers was determined to launch the country's third dedicated service in Kent. In November 1989, the South East Thames Air Ambulance (as it was then known) was born, flying its first mission a few weeks later. In 2007 it combined with Surrey and Sussex to double their resources and became the Kent, Surrey and Sussex Air Ambulance Trust. In 2013, the KSSAAT were the first non-hospital-based service to carry blood in order to perform transfusions at the scene of an accident or medical emergency. The charity's headquarters is located at Rochester Airport, with its three aircraft – an MD 902 Explorer and two AW169s – hangared and maintained at Redhill Aerodrome, enabling the charity to provide 24/7 operations reaching any part of their region within 25 minutes.

Lincolnshire and Nottinghamshire Air Ambulance Charitable Trust (LNAACT)

After three years of planning and fundraising, the Lincolnshire Air Ambulance first became operational in 1994. At the start, its helicopter, an ex-police Bölkow aircraft, only flew when there was sufficient income – meaning it was often grounded for months at a time while fundraising took place. However, in 1995 a two-year sponsorship deal with the *Lincolnshire Standard* newspaper group allowed the service to fly 365 days a year. A year later the service was extended to cover Nottinghamshire with a sponsorship deal from the *Nottingham Post*. LNAACT is currently in the process of transitioning to a full 24 hours a day, seven days a week HEMS

RIGHT Lincolnshire and Nottinghamshire Air Ambulance Charitable Trust is transitioning to a 24/7 service with its AW169. *(LNAACT)*

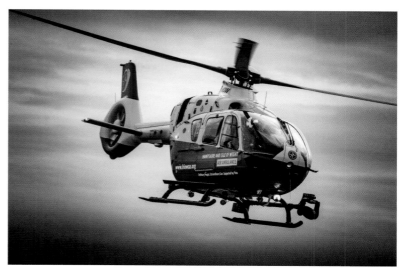

ABOVE Hampshire and Isle of Wight Air Ambulance operates an Airbus H135 helicopter from its base in Thruxton. *(Simon Heron)*

BELOW Kent, Surrey and Sussex Air Ambulance Trust operates a 24/7 service with its two AW169s and an MD 902 Explorer. *(KSAAT)*

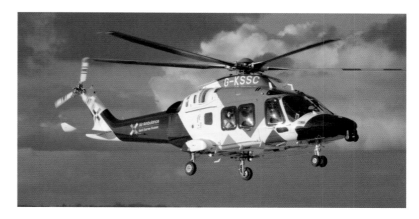

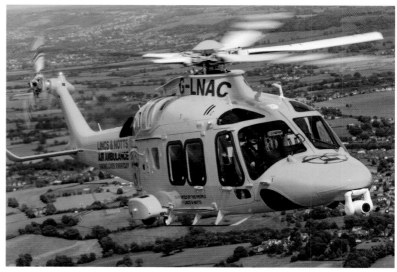

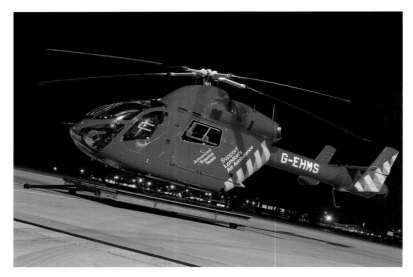

ABOVE **The two MD 902 Explorer helicopters of London's Air Ambulance fly only during daylight hours, with an average flight time of six minutes.** *(London's Air Ambulance)*

service in 2019, making it one of only three air ambulance charities in the UK to operate a helicopter 24 hours a day. It flies an AW169 and also operates a rapid response vehicle.

London's Air Ambulance Charity

The principle of a doctor-paramedic advanced trauma team was pioneered by London's Air Ambulance. On Christmas Eve 1993, the crew performed the world's first successful open heart surgery at the roadside and the service is now considered a leader in pre-hospital care in the UK and abroad. In 2010, the service

started operating 24/7 and in 2014 it appointed the UK's first patient liaison nurse for trauma patients. London's Air Ambulance operates two MD 902 Explorer helicopters, which were specially selected for their suitability in an urban environment; they are small with no tail rotor, which allows the service to operate safely in an area as complicated and congested as London. They also have a fleet of five rapid response vehicles, which are used at night and during adverse weather conditions.

Mid Anglia General Practitioner Accident Service (Magpas) Air Ambulance

Established in 1971, Magpas was one of the UK's first emergency medical charities, founded by two GPs from Cambridgeshire, Dr Neville Silverston MBE and Dr Derek Cracknell MBE. They worked together to create the Mid Anglia General Practitioner Accident Service (what is now known as Magpas Air Ambulance), a voluntary service of more than 100 GPs around Cambridgeshire who could be called upon, day or night, to treat patients at the scene of road accidents. Responding in their own cars, Magpas brought medical care to the scene of incidents, treating patients there and then and giving them a much better chance of survival and recovery.

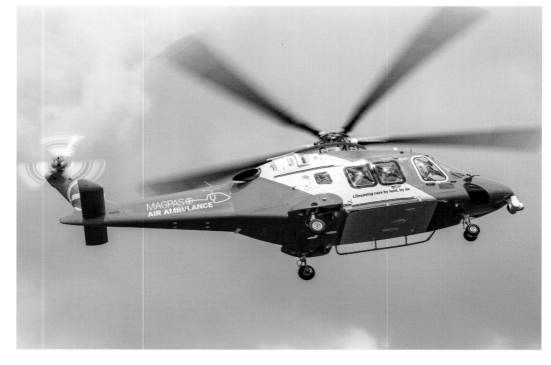

RIGHT **Magpas was one of the UK's first emergency medical charities, founded in 1971. It now offers pioneering training to doctors and paramedics.** *(Magpas)*

This still remains at the heart of the charity today, and now Magpas Air Ambulance offer pioneering training to expert doctors and paramedics to bring advanced, lifesaving care to seriously ill and injured patients across the East of England and beyond, via an air ambulance and two rapid response vehicles, 24/7.

Midlands Air Ambulance Charity (MAAC)

MAAC operates and funds three air ambulances covering six Midlands counties, including Gloucestershire, Herefordshire, Shropshire, Staffordshire, Worcestershire and the West Midlands. Funded entirely by donations, the charity relies on support from local people and businesses to raise the £9 million needed to undertake on average 2,000 missions every year. Since 1991, MAAC has responded to over 50,000 missions, making it one of the busiest air ambulance services in the UK. The charity responds to some of the most traumatic incidents, including cardiac arrests, road traffic collisions and falls.

North West Air Ambulance Charity (NWAA)

Founded in 1999, North West Air Ambulance Charity (NWAA) operates three

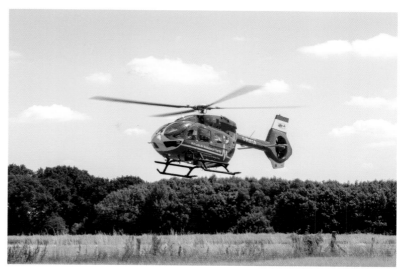

EC135 helicopters and two rapid response vehicles from its two bases in Blackpool and Barton. Two of the aircraft have a twin-paramedic clinical crew, while the third has a paramedic and doctor on board. Between them, the three helicopters attend a total of around 2,000 missions every year. Serving Cumbria, Lancashire, Greater Manchester, Merseyside and Cheshire, NWAA uses a range of fundraising techniques in addition to operating 11 charity retail outlets across the North West to help it to raise funds in excess of £9m per year.

ABOVE Midlands Air Ambulance Charity operates three aircraft, which cover six Midlands counties. *(MAAC)*

BELOW North West Air Ambulance Charity operates three EC135 helicopters and two rapid response vehicles. *(NWAA)*

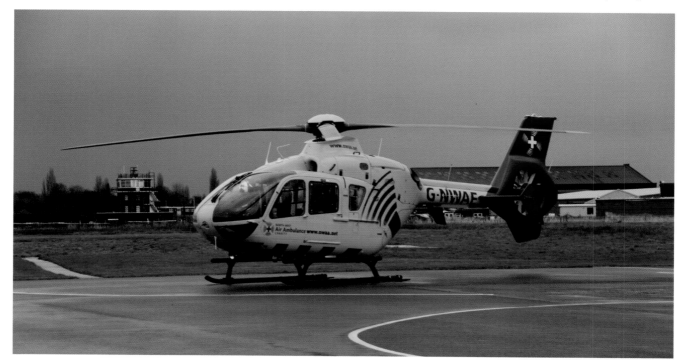

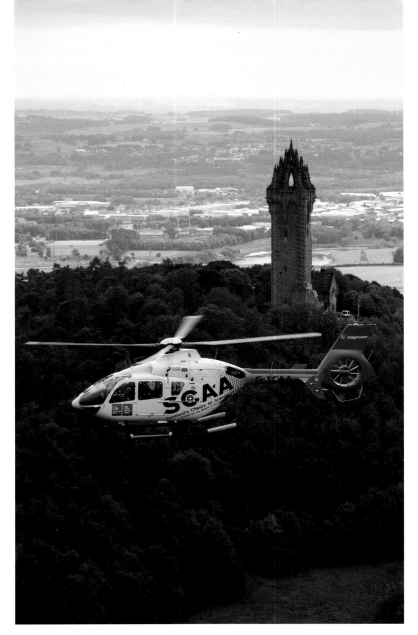

Scotland's Charity Air Ambulance (SCAA)

SCAA launched in May 2013. SCAA forms an integral part of Scotland's frontline emergency response network, responding to trauma incidents and medical emergencies across the country, covering an area of more than 30,000 square miles and serving a population of over five million. Based at Perth Airport, the helicopter can reach 90% of Scotland's population within 25 minutes. Following a £6m fundraising drive, SCAAs intend to launch a second air ambulance helicopter, based in Aberdeen.

Thames Valley Air Ambulance (TVAA)

TVAA is an independent healthcare provider of advanced critical care within Berkshire, Buckinghamshire and Oxfordshire, bringing the expertise, equipment and treatment of the hospital to the patient. From its base at RAF Benson in South Oxfordshire, TVAA can reach any point in Berkshire, Oxfordshire and Buckinghamshire within 15 minutes using its Airbus H135 and was the first HEMS unit

LEFT The EC135 of Scotland's Charity Air Ambulance flying over the National Wallace Monument, Stirling. *(SCAA)*

BELOW Thames Valley Air Ambulance operates an Airbus H135 and four Emergency Response Vehicles, which roam the areas where the helicopter struggles to gain quick access. *(TVAA)*

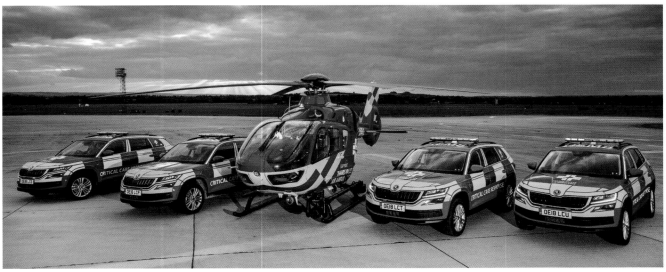

in the country to carry plasma on board for critically injured trauma patients. TVAA works in partnership with Hampshire and Isle of Wight Air Ambulance to provide a night-flying service from 19:00h to 02:00h every day, with the charities taking it in turns to cover the whole of the South Central region and the Isle of Wight.

The Air Ambulance Service (TAAS)

Covering Warwickshire, Northamptonshire, Derbyshire, Leicestershire and Rutland, TAAS started out in 2003 as the Warwickshire & Northamptonshire Air Ambulance, with sister service the Derbyshire, Leicestershire and Rutland Air Ambulance launching in 2008. The two services were brought together under the umbrella name of TAAS in 2011. Its two AW109 helicopters cover trauma and medical emergencies over an area of 3,850 square miles, covering many of the UK's major road networks, including the M1, M6, M69 and M42. This vital service is undertaken by aircraft during the daylight hours and rapid response vehicles during night-time hours.

TAAS also operates The Children's Air Ambulance (TCAA), which was launched in 2012 and is the only dedicated paediatric and neo-natal national transfer service. The TCAA works collaboratively with nine specialist neonatal and paediatric Clinical Partner Teams (CPTs) across the country to transfer critically ill children to specialist care, to move specialist clinical teams to district hospitals to treat critically ill children and to repatriate children back to their local hospital following specialist care. TCAA has worked collaboratively with the nine CPTs to design the aircraft interior layout and equipment, and since September 2018 has expanded its fleet to two aircraft using state-of-the-art AW169 helicopters, which have an increased cabin size and enhanced capabilities from both clinical and aviation aspects.

Wales Air Ambulance Charitable Trust (WAACT)

St David's Day 2001 saw the launch of the Wales Air Ambulance. With four aircraft operating from airbases in Caernarfon, Llanelli, Welshpool and Cardiff, it is now the largest air ambulance operation in the UK, with annual

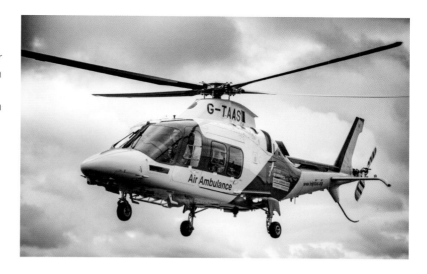

ABOVE The Air Ambulance Service covers five counties and also operates The Children's Air Ambulance. *(TAAS)*

BELOW Wales Air Ambulance is the largest air ambulance operation in the UK, with four aircraft operating from airbases throughout the country. *(WAACT)*

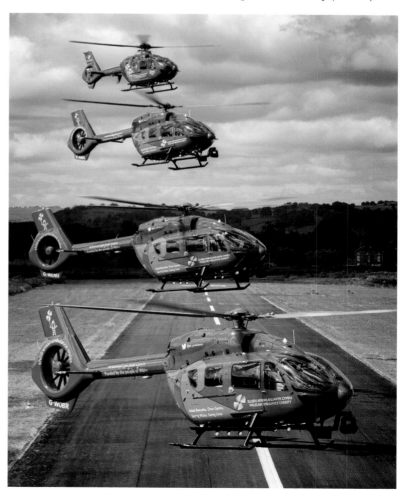

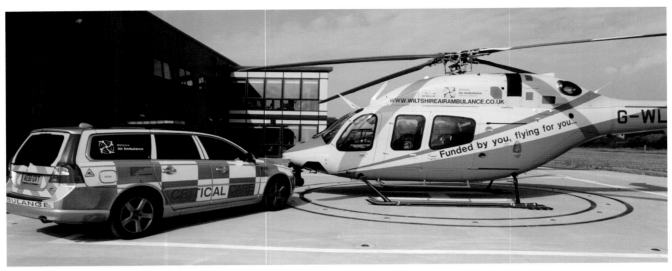

running costs of more than £6.5 million. Alongside WAACT'S consultant-led HEMS service, it also operates the Children's Wales Air Ambulance. This is a specialist division of the charity, with a dedicated transfer helicopter providing expert care and transport for paediatric and neonatal patients in Wales.

Wiltshire Air Ambulance (WAA)

Wiltshire Air Ambulance started operations in March 1990. The charity shared a helicopter with Wiltshire Police for 24 years and started operating as a stand-alone air ambulance in January 2015, using a Bell 429 helicopter. WAA moved into its new airbase at Outmarsh, Semington, near Melksham, in May 2018, with the official opening by the charity's patron, HRH The Duchess of Cornwall, in December 2018. From this central site the helicopter can reach anywhere in the county within 11 minutes, while the charity also has two rapid response vehicles to attend incidents by road.

Yorkshire Air Ambulance Charity (YAAC)

The largest county in England, Yorkshire's topography includes remote, rural and densely populated areas as well as major motorways and road networks. Yorkshire Air Ambulance (YAA) provides its life-saving service to five million people, covering four million acres of Yorkshire with its two H145 helicopters, based between Nostell Air Support Unit near Wakefield and RAF Topcliffe, near Thirsk. YAA currently attends some 1,000 incidents a year and to

keep both aircraft maintained and in the air costs £4.4m annually. The charity was set up in 2000 and added its second air ambulance in 2007. The service features in the Really TV series, *Helicopter ER*.

UK AIR AMBULANCE SERVICES: LAUNCH DATES	
Service	**Year**
Cornwall Air Ambulance Trust	1987
London's Air Ambulance Charity	1989
Kent, Surrey and Sussex Air Ambulance Trust	1989
Wiltshire Air Ambulance	1990
Great North Air Ambulance Service	1991
Midlands Air Ambulance Charity	1991
Devon Air Ambulance Trust	1992
Lincolnshire and Nottinghamshire Air Ambulance Charitable Trust	1994
Magpas Air Ambulance	1997
Essex & Herts Air Ambulance Trust	1998
North West Air Ambulance Charity	1999
Dorset and Somerset Air Ambulance	2000
East Anglian Air Ambulance	2000
Yorkshire Air Ambulance Charity	2000
Thames Valley Air Ambulance	2000
Wales Air Ambulance Charitable Trust	2001
The Air Ambulance Service	2003
Great Western Air Ambulance Charity	2007
Hampshire and Isle of Wight Air Ambulance	2007
Scotland's Charity Air Ambulance	2013
Air Ambulance Northern Ireland	2017

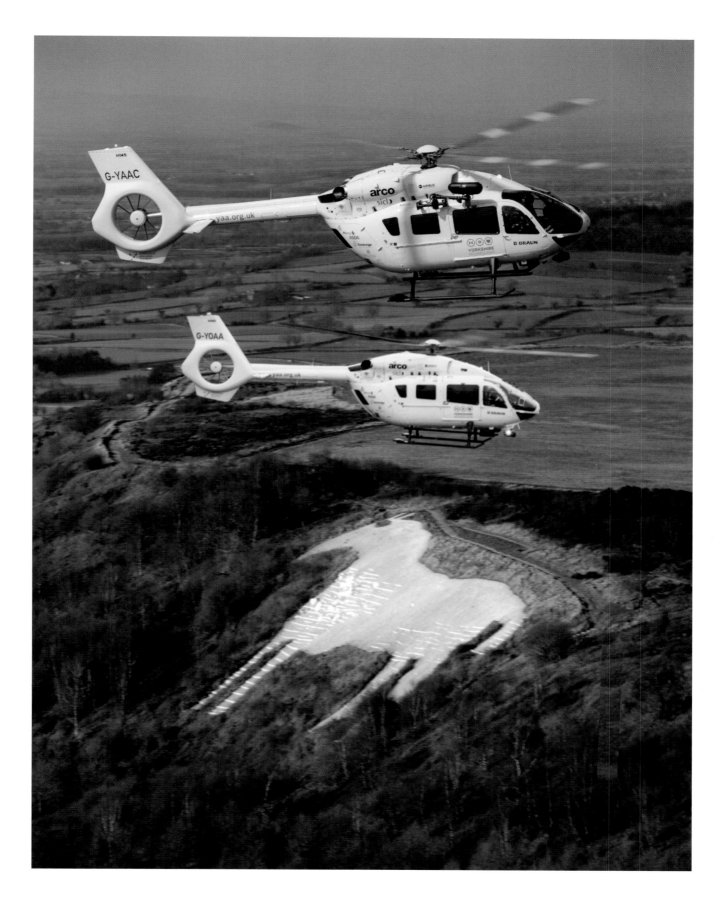

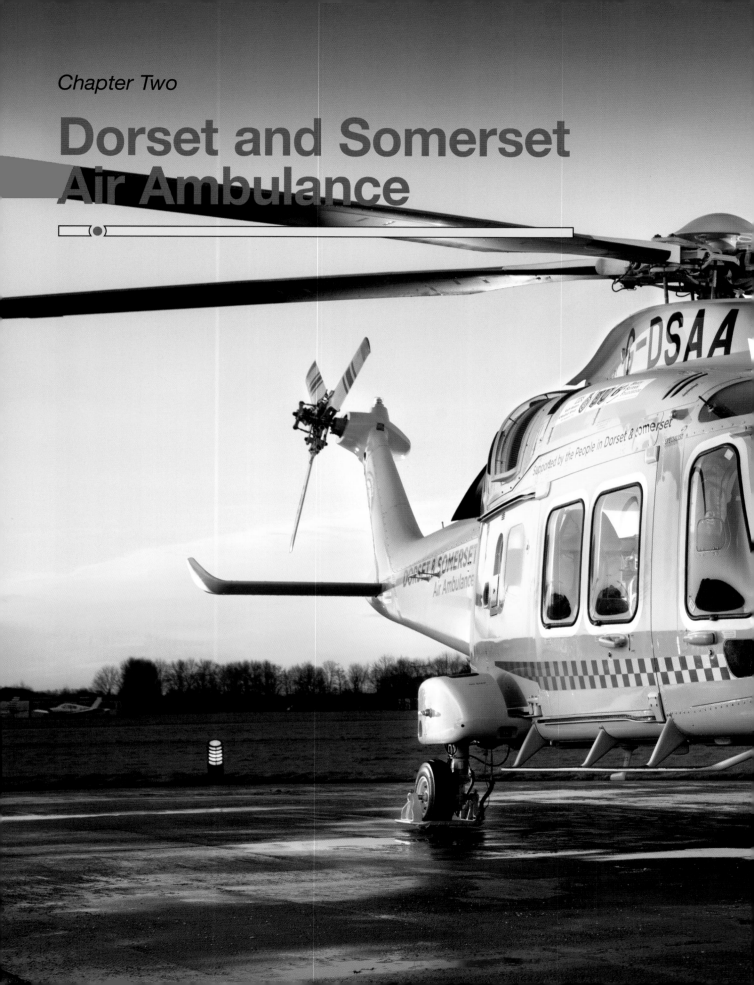

Chapter Two

Dorset and Somerset
Air Ambulance

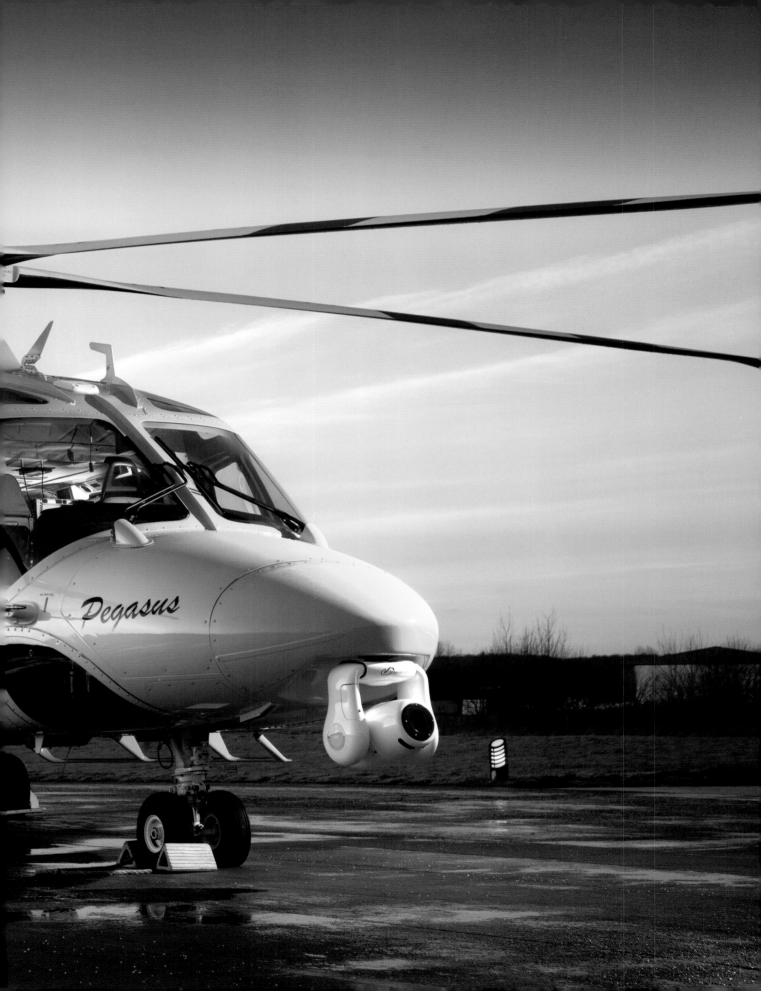

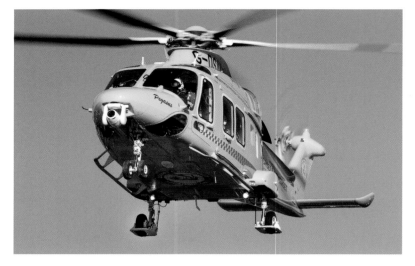

Why the DSAA?

When it came to selecting a specific UK air ambulance service to focus on, it was difficult to choose between them. They all have different operational methods, different clinical models – even different aircraft. Where to start? As it was impossible to select an ambulance service based on merit, we instead opted to start our research based on geography.

Haynes's headquarters is located near Yeovil in Somerset, close to the Dorset border, so when planning for this manual began, it seemed logical to start by making contact with the local air ambulance service. Launched in 2000, Dorset and Somerset Air Ambulance (DSAA) was one of the first air ambulances to use the AW169 helicopter in operational service, which reinforced the local connection, as Leonardo, manufacturer of the AW169, also has its UK base in Somerset.

DSAA is one of 21 registered air ambulance charities in the UK, with a remit to provide relief from sickness and injury for the people of both counties. The air ambulance is tasked

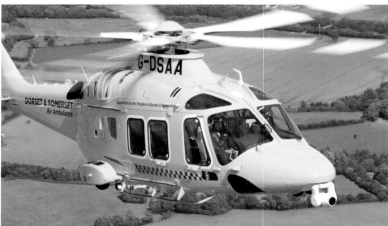

LEFT AND BELOW Launched in 2000, the DSAA was one of the first air ambulances to use the AW169 helicopter in operational service. *(Leonardo Helicopters/Simon Pryor)*

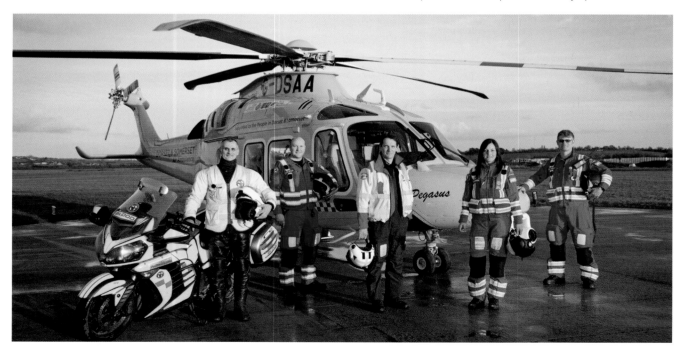

as part of the normal 999 emergency process by a dedicated Helicopter Emergency Medical Service (HEMS) desk located at Ambulance Control. Situated at Henstridge Airfield on the Dorset/Somerset border, the service is operational for 19 hours a day, 365 days a year and can reach any point in the two counties in less than 20 minutes. The helicopter can, if required, then take a patient to the nearest specialist medical or trauma centre in the South West within a further 20 minutes.

Mission and vision

In the early days of air ambulances, their main advantage was the speed with which they could reach a patient and lift them to hospital. Modern-day air ambulances offer far more than that, bringing expert skills and expert decision-making to the patient as quickly as possible – effectively bringing the hospital to the roadside. Each DSAA mission is attended by a critical care team, consisting of one doctor and at least one Critical Care Practitioner, sometimes two depending on the time of day. This enhanced level of care represents a paradigm shift in pre-hospital emergency medicine: bringing the intensive care unit and resuscitation department to the patient's side within a matter of minutes.

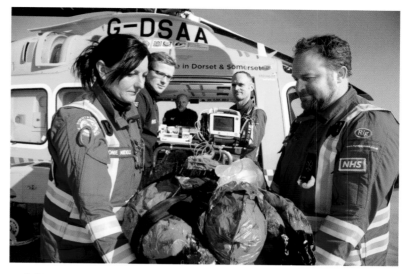

DSAA's vision centres on three key aspects: clinical excellence, efficiency and effectiveness, and financial security. It aims to provide the maximum benefit to patients by delivering an air ambulance service to the South West region that conforms to these three basic principles.

Origins

For the counties of Dorset and Somerset, having an air ambulance is a relatively recent thing. In 2000, a grant from a fund established by the Automobile Association (AA) was distributed to existing air ambulances in the

ABOVE Each DSAA mission is attended by a critical care team of one doctor and at least one Critical Care Practitioner.

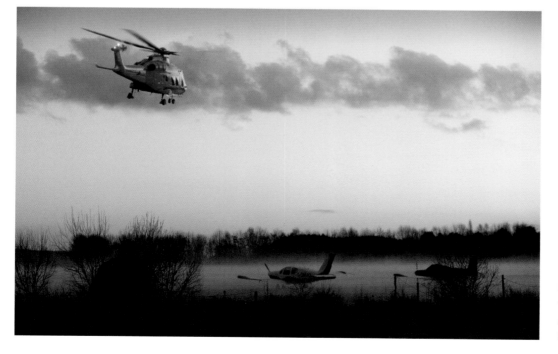

LEFT DSAA operates from Henstridge Airfield, on the Dorset/ Somerset border.

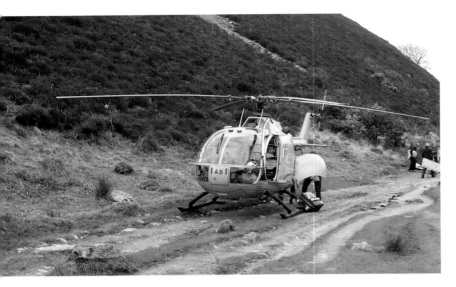

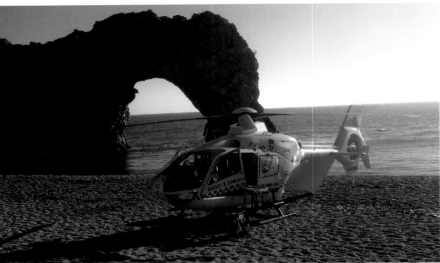

UK and to those organisations that required funds to start. In setting up the fund, the AA had planned to emulate the German system, where its equivalent organisation, the German Automobile Club (Allgemeiner Deutscher Automobil-Club or ADAC) was operating the first air ambulances in Germany. However, this endeavour proved more challenging than the AA had anticipated, given that the fund had been started after the call for air ambulances had already begun and a number of community initiatives already existed.

The AA ended up with a fund of some £14 million and, rather than operate air ambulances itself, decided instead to disperse the money to existing air ambulances for development and to aspirant air ambulances to get them started. At around the same time in Dorset and Somerset, there was a transition going on in the region's ambulance service – Dorset Ambulance Service had joined the Western Ambulance Service, forming the South Western Ambulance Service. Having seen air ambulance services start up in Cornwall in 1987 and in Devon five years later, the late Sir Brian Kenny (1934–2017) and a group of others felt it was time that the remaining two West Country counties should have their own.

The Dorset and Somerset Air Ambulance charity was registered in December 1999, with its official start in January 2000. The charity entered into an arrangement with Bond Air Services and launched its service in March 2000, with the AA funding effectively covering the first few years of operation.

The first aircraft operated by DSAA was a Bölkow 105 (BO 105) helicopter. A launch ceremony at Sherborne Castle in Dorset saw

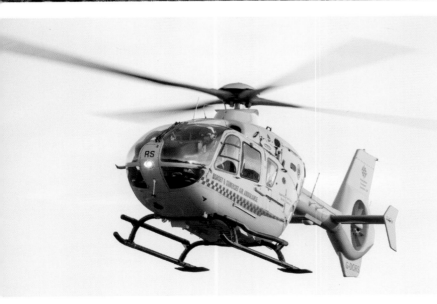

the BO 105 fly in through heavy rain, escorted by colleagues from Cornwall and Devon. The aircraft carried a crew of two paramedics and a pilot, and would operate on every day of the year during the hours of daylight. It would be airborne within three minutes of a call being received, reach the scene of the incident within a maximum of 20y minutes and be at the nearest hospital within a further ten minutes.

On 21 March, its first day of operations, the service came online at 08.00h and was tasked with its first mission within the hour. By the end of its first year of service, DSAA had completed 617 missions over the two counties, transporting 285 casualties to hospital or to one of the regional trauma centres. The missions took place almost equally between Dorset and Somerset; nearly half of all missions were to road accidents, with the remainder being split (in descending order) between collapses, recreational accidents, falls and work accidents. Lives were saved in numerous missions where the speed of the response and the subsequent delivery to hospital by the air ambulance enabled the A&E specialists to get to work sooner than they would have if the patient had been delivered by traditional means. In many cases, the same speed of delivery resulted in a faster and fuller recovery with a reduction in the length of hospital stay,

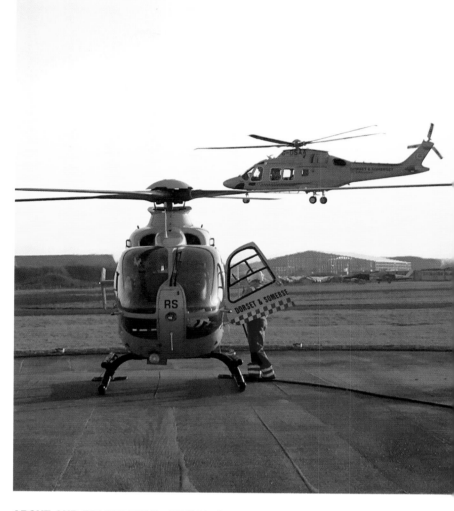

ABOVE AND BELOW DSAA's AW169 helicopter entered operational service on 12 June 2017.

DSAA: CORE VALUES

- **Teamwork:** Aircrew, business partners, staff, trustees, volunteers and the community – one team.
- **Respect:** We treat everyone with the highest degree of dignity, equality and trust.
- **Accountability:** We take responsibility for our performance in all of our decisions and actions.
- **Integrity:** We demonstrate honesty and fairness in every action that we take.
- **Innovation:** We anticipate change and capitalise on the many opportunities that arise.

These values will be at the heart of every decision and action.

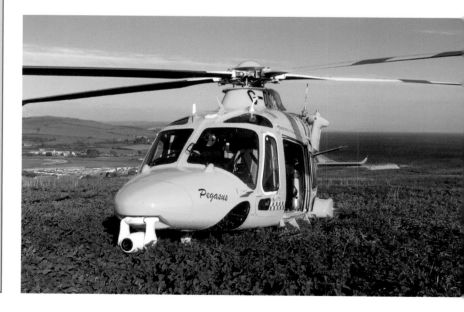

providing an added bonus both to the patient and to the NHS.

Since its launch, DSAA has flown in excess of 12,500 missions. The service now operates for 19 hours a day, from 07.00h–02.00h, using two vital resources: an AW169 helicopter and two Skoda Kodiaq critical care cars.

Management and operational structure

The charity is based in Somerset, with an office in Wellington and the air ambulance based at Henstridge Airfield, near the Dorset border. Geoff Jarvis, owner of Henstridge Airfield, is a staunch supporter of DSAA. As well as providing its hangar and helipad, his consideration for the charity in day-to-day airfield matters has ensured that its operations, aircraft arrivals and departures are as efficient as they can be. Geoff facilitates DSAA's fundraising and public engagement events and often raises funds for the charity by organising his own events. He is also a real advocate for DSAA with other airfield users.

DSAA is controlled by a board of trustees, whose job it is to ensure the charity is run properly and effectively, and that it meets its overall purpose. The board comprises a chairperson and up to 12 trustees; each one is appointed in accordance with the charity's constitution and has responsibilities that are set within clearly defined and approved terms of reference. Trustees help to shape the long-term direction of the charity and between them, they bring a broad range of skills and experience in a number of areas, including healthcare, aviation, law, business, finance, military service, charities and local affairs. Representatives from Specialist Aviation Services and South Western Ambulance Service NHS Foundation Trust (SWASFT) also attend board meetings as and when required, to provide additional operational advice.

In total, there are 13 full-time equivalent administrative staff employed by the charity, including the CEO, a fundraising manager, a communications manager, a charity manager (job share between two individuals), a compliance officer and a lottery manager. Considering the charity had an £8.5 million turnover in 2018, this is a small number, reflecting one of the organisation's core principles: efficiency.

The air ambulance operational crew is a team made up of pilots, an engineer and, of course, clinical staff. DSAA's four pilots and engineer are hired, trained and provided by Specialist Aviation Services, which operates the aircraft for the charity. The pilots undergo a careful selection procedure because air ambulance flights are typically more challenging than regular, non-emergency flight services. Each pilot has a great deal of experience in low-level operations and instrument flying, and one of them is nominated as the unit chief pilot.

DSAA's clinical team includes 28 full-time equivalent operational members, two patient and family liaison nurses, a training/education facilitator and an administrator. The operational crew includes intensive care, emergency medicine and anaesthetic physicians and Critical Care Practitioners (paramedics or nurses). Part of their role includes assisting the pilot with the safe operation of the aircraft and they undergo specific training to assist with navigation and operation of some of the aircraft's systems.

A critical care team, consisting of at least one doctor and one Critical Care Practitioner, is

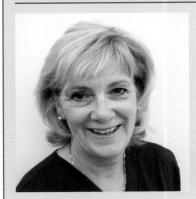

present for each mission. There are 14 full-time equivalent Critical Care Practitioners (the term used to describe the multi-disciplinary nature of the team members; a mix of nurses and paramedics). The doctors are all at consultant grade, with either an emergency medicine, anaesthesia or intensive care background. All the Critical Care Cractitioners are employed by or under contract to SWASFT and are seconded to DSAA through a service level agreement.

In recent years, clinicians have also joined from further afield, broadening the skills and experience of the team. At the time of writing, Medical Lead Phil Hyde is the senior doctor and Operational Lead Paul Owen is the senior practitioner. Paul is DSAA's longest-serving staff member, having joined in 2004.

All clinical care practitioners have either completed or are going through an MSc advanced paramedic practice (critical care) qualification, with varying modules depending on where they are in their progress. DSAA supports all its clinicians (whether practitioners or doctors) in their further professional development. All are encouraged to complete the Diploma in Immediate Medical Care (DIMC) of the Faculty of Pre-Hospital Care of the Royal College of Surgeons of Edinburgh. Four of the team have also achieved the Fellowship in Immediate Medical Care (FIMC). Fourteen of the team are qualified as pre-hospital examiners for the Royal College.

Clinical model

DSAA's fundamental belief is to put the patient right at the centre of everything and to do whatever is in their best interest. It is important for the public and other emergency services on the ground to know that an air ambulance doesn't just mean a faster taxi-ride to the right destination, but that the skills and expertise of its crew bring added diagnostic and technical skills to the scene and en route to hospital.

When it started out, the service's original twin-paramedic model of operation was pretty much the standard of the time and changed very little for many years. The principle was to get to the patient as quickly as possible, carry out an immediate

CHIEF EXECUTIVE OFFICER: BILL SIVEWRIGHT

Day-to-day operations are overseen by Chief Executive Officer Bill Sivewright. A qualified helicopter pilot and British army veteran, Bill spent three decades serving in a variety of staff officer and flying appointments, before assuming roles at NATO and Joint Helicopter Command. In 2004/05 he commanded the Joint Helicopter Force in Iraq before returning to the UK to serve in the UK Joint Helicopter Command and ultimately as assistant director of Army Aviation and Regimental Colonel of the Army Air Corps.

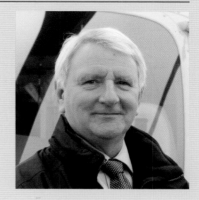

ABOVE Bill Sivewright, **DSAA chief executive.**

Bill joined DSAA in 2010 and is responsible for the overall operation of the air ambulance, its finances, facilities and staff and the service provided to the people of Dorset and Somerset, in line with the policy, direction and guidance set by the board. Bill is answerable not only to the board, but also to the people of Dorset and Somerset. He spends a fair amount of time out of the office meeting the public and giving talks. 'Quite a lot of what we do is complex and needs quite careful explanation,' he says. 'I enjoy getting out there and presenting to the public because it enables me to clarify aspects of what we do and why we do it. It also allows me to get valuable feedback from our supporters.'

assessment, stabilise them and package them for transportation to hospital.

However, over the past two decades, what was initially a single model for delivery has developed into a multitude of models. Variances in aviation and clinical governance, ownership of aircraft and employment of clinical staff are all now part of the mix. Over the years, there have been cries for a more consistent, national approach. 'Economies of scale in procurement and ease of understanding for bodies such as the Department of Health and the Civil Aviation Authority are two good arguments for taking that line,' says Bill Sivewright, CEO. 'However, it fails to recognise why such variability exists in the first place. The way we operate is subject to a number of variable factors. Geography is an obvious one but the key factor is that of the NHS environment in which we sit. Funding,

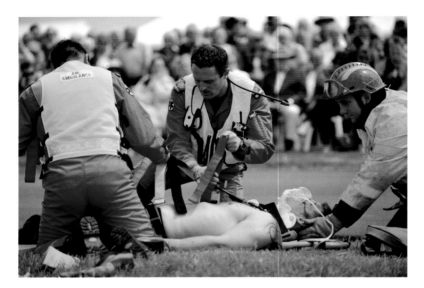

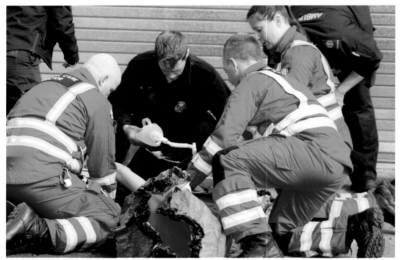

ABOVE DSAA's fundamental belief is to put the patient right at the centre of everything.

RIGHT Farhad Islam (Izzy) was the first doctor to fly with DSAA and was responsible for creating the university-accredited education programme for paramedics.

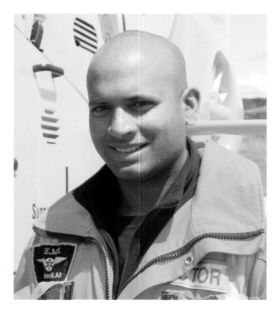

staffing, logistics and priorities for categories of care are all subject to local influences and shape the environment that we as an air ambulance operate in.'

Education: a new tier of paramedic

In 2011, DSAA started looking for ways to further develop its clinical capability. At that time, the charity was still strategically committed to a twin-paramedic model of delivery, so its only course of action was to 'upskill' its paramedics. It was decided that the best way forward would be for the crew to undertake post-graduate-level education, which would provide them with a qualification they could take with them anywhere. 'The way to move forward from our twin-paramedic model was to firstly help those paramedics be as good as they could possibly be,' explains Bill. Increasing a paramedic's patient assessment skills, widening their knowledge of drugs, improving their diagnostic abilities, advancing their management of pain and becoming better at clinical decision-making would all be key factors in continuing to provide clinical excellence to patients.

From the outset, DSAA had been gathering data on what difference doctors might be able to make to its service and, two years in, it was decided that having a doctor on every mission could make a vast difference, so DSAA chose to develop this further.

Farhad Islam (Izzy) was the first doctor to fly with DSAA, joining in 2007 on a part-time basis, having just started as an emergency medicine consultant at the Royal Bournemouth & Poole Hospitals. As a junior doctor learning his trade, Izzy had attended the Paddington rail crash and was amazed at the service provided by the London HEMS team. He geared his whole career from then on to make sure he became an air ambulance doctor, studying emergency medicine and then moving to Auckland to work with the Westpac Air Ambulance. When he returned to London and finished his emergency physician training, he ended up working a nine-month HEMS Registrar and Physician Response Unit post with London's Air Ambulance.

During his time as a HEMS doctor, Izzy realised that most air ambulance paramedics did not get much recognition for what they could do. They were often more experienced than doctors, simply because of the nature of the cases they were seeing, yet they were unable to perform the same range of clinical procedures. After joining DSAA, Izzy was determined to change this and was responsible for initiating a project that would see DSAA fund a unique, university-accredited education programme for eight paramedics.

As the first doctor to join DSAA, Izzy's arrival had marked a culture change for the crew, who were used to operating with paramedics alone. Adding doctors to the mix needed to be managed sensitively – in other HEMS operations, with doctor-led services, paramedics sometimes play a secondary role and it was important for Izzy to make it clear that the intention here was to operate as a team. DSAA's paramedics already had a wealth of skills and experience in pre-hospital medicine and the plan was to recognise this formally.

The result was a three-year MSc Advanced Paramedic Practice (critical care) qualification, funded by DSAA and run in partnership with the University of Hertfordshire, the SWASFT and a number of NHS Hospital Trusts across the region. This knowledge-based, practical master's course would provide the paramedics with many of the competencies that doctors already had, enabling them to work more effectively as a team.

The concept itself wasn't new in the sense that nurses around the country had been trained up to be practitioners in various specialties. However, Izzy's plan was to design a bespoke critical care paramedic course to equip paramedics with more practical skills, clinical knowledge and critical-thinking skills. It would give them both the theoretical knowledge and practical skills for life-saving procedures such as opening up a temporary airway through the neck or relieving a tension pneumothorax (build-up of pressure in the lung). It would provide operating skills, such as the ability to perform a thoracotomy (opening a patient's chest at the scene, using specialist equipment). Paramedics would learn about the advantages, the side effects and the governance related to giving blood as well as how to administer it. They would also develop decision-making skills,

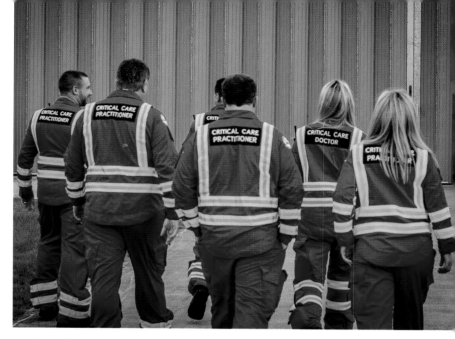

such as when to make certain interventions and when not to, and learn about the benefits and pitfalls of administering particular drugs to the critically injured or critically ill body. And, crucially, the degree would teach analytical and evaluation skills so that each paramedic would understand how to improve the service, analysing and critically appraising the latest drugs or pieces of medical equipment and deciding whether to implement use of them.

To set things in motion, DSAA had to recruit a group of senior critical care doctors to come and work with the paramedics, although not many doctors were trained in HEMS in Dorset and Somerset at this stage. What was soon apparent was that this was very much a two-way learning process, with the doctors learning just as much from the paramedics. Paramedics, for example, are well versed in scene management and are used to leadership at the roadside – dealing with the police, the public, fire and rescue and other professionals on scene. They are experienced in dealing with multiple casualties at a scene or treating patients in challenging locations, such as a car that has rolled over – whereas most doctors were more used to operating within a relatively safe hospital environment.

For some of the paramedics, a number of years had passed since they had undergone formal education, so some encouragement was needed before they felt able to embark on a master's-level degree. A training needs analysis was undertaken, based on what the paramedics already knew and what they

ABOVE The three-year MSc Advanced Paramedic Practice (Critical Care) qualification provides paramedics with many of the competencies that doctors already have. *(John Emery)*

needed to learn. Additionally, DSAA needed to identify the skill set that could reasonably be expected of them, taking into account the imminent changes in healthcare, the development of major trauma centres and the regionalisation of acute stroke and cardiac care.

Service level agreements (SLAs) were set up with local hospitals and consultants were employed for three days a week to help train the paramedics. In parallel, a way of recording and measuring the impact of the project was designed to help support and sustain the initiative.

One unique element of the whole programme, which started in 2013, was the fact that the education and training was largely delivered on-site at the charity's Henstridge airbase and not in the university classroom. This enabled mentoring both on land and in the air. Given the nature of the degree, it was more easily delivered in the workplace, so part of the education and training was based at the university, part at the airbase and part of it online. Hospitals also provided short placements for the paramedics, to help them gain first-hand experience of conditions and treatments that they may not necessarily have encountered

with the air ambulance. This involved practical, on-the-job learning with a senior clinician, either an anaesthetist, an intensivist (a physician who specialises in critically ill patients) or an emergency physician. To gain competencies, the paramedics spent time in intensive care units, in theatres observing operations, and in the emergency departments of district hospitals and major trauma centres.

Regular clinical governance and training days gave paramedics the opportunity to work on real-life scenarios, using state-of-the-art equipment and training tools. The collaborative training events allowed paramedics to share their knowledge and experience with other clinicians on topics such as advanced haemorrhage control techniques and resuscitative surgery within the pre-hospital care environment.

The culture of shared learning and inter-disciplinary teamwork was recorded in detail on two new databases. These captured all the lectures, articles, education and competencies that had been achieved in order to deliver effective governance, improve communications and measure impact.

The investment made by DSAA undoubtedly

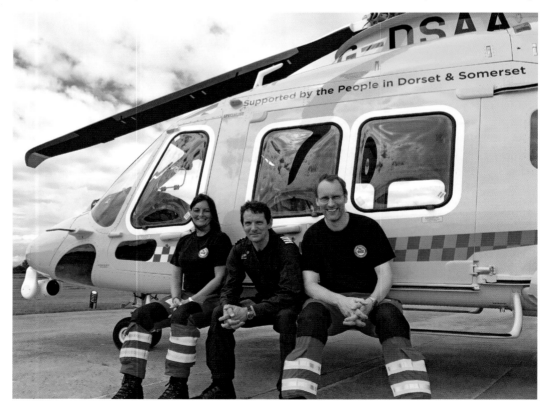

RIGHT Education and training is largely delivered on-site at Henstridge Airfield. Pictured: DSAA crew members Leonie German, Phil Merritt and Jeremy Reid.

improved the quality of care being delivered to patients across the South West of England. DSAA paramedics, who the service calls Critical Care Practitioners, are now able to provide new drug treatments and procedures, all within the pre-hospital care environment. This includes safe delivery of controlled drugs like ketamine to act as either a sedative or an analgesic. Paramedics now understand the pathology and disease of trauma and critical care, which helps to underpin the decisions they make regarding drugs and treatment. They do not study this to the same in-depth biochemical and physiological level as a doctor, but in the field working within the team, that level of detail is unnecessary. They also have skills of diagnosis that a regular paramedic doesn't have. If confronted with a head injury, for example, they know what could happen to the brain, what signs to look for and they have the ability to recognise when disease is progressing and know how to act and how urgently.

The master's degree also had a number of applications in the wider world. During the final year of the course, each student takes one particular subject and critically appraises it in great depth; for example, exploring the use of ultrasound in the pre-hospital field, or the use of blood products, or how to improve tasking of air ambulance crews. As well as helping with the paramedic's day-to-day practice, this research will help to further an area of care and knowledge that will be of benefit to the whole medical community.

Another consequence was the establishment of a new tier of paramedic within SWASFT, the 'critical care paramedic'. Following the success of this project, several other air ambulance charities and trusts are looking to emulate the programme or use the framework to help develop their own service.

Having established the education programme and started to deliver it, it became clear that there was a lot more that could be achieved. 'It was like lighting a blue touch paper,' says Bill. 'Within a very short time, it was apparent that the enthusiasm of the paramedics for the exposure they were getting to high-grade consultant mentorship in real-world experience, coupled with the consultants' complete buy-in, was delivering much more than the sum of the parts.'

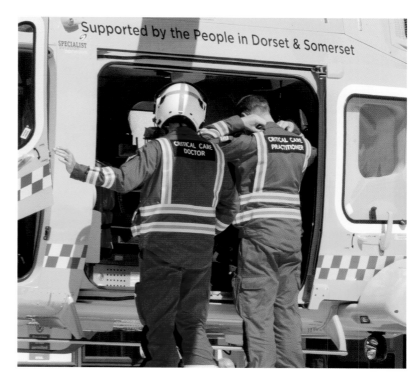

While DSAA was not the first air ambulance organisation to consider using doctors as part of its team, the charity felt that its team ethos would be better served by the doctor being an implicit part of the team rather than an explicit one. In 2015 it therefore embarked on a restructuring exercise, which saw the formal creation of a critical care team.

Critical care teams

O ver the past few years, air ambulance medicine has been moving towards a critical care focused delivery, which has been supported by the creation of the PHEM

ABOVE The learning process was very much two-way, with the doctors learning just as much from the paramedics.

BELOW In 2016, DSAA started providing a full critical care service, consisting of at least one Critical Care Practitioner and one critical care doctor on each mission.

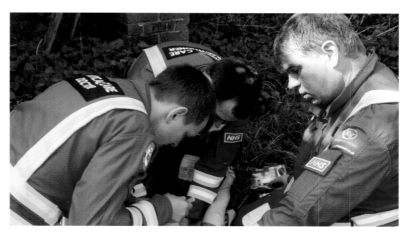

Paul became DSAA's Operational Lead in 2007 and is responsible for the operational running of the service. Reporting to South Western Ambulance Service NHS Foundation Trust (SWASFT) and the DSAA Executive Board and senior management team, his role is to ensure smooth day-to-day running of the aircraft, as well as working closely with the DSAA Medical Lead Phil Hyde to improve governance of DSAA clinical operations. Paul provides support and leadership to DSAA clinical team members, developing systems and operational structures that enable them to safely adhere to SWASFT governance requirements (all paramedics are employed by SWASFT, which oversees governance and training records). He undertakes regular clinical case reviews, manages the team's continued professional development and works with clinicians, hospitals and networks across the South of England to improve patient care and pathways.

On a day-to-day basis, as well as regularly covering shifts, Paul is responsible for organising shifts, overseeing the drugs and medical equipment, dealing with problems if they arise, carrying out welfare checks and liaising with SWASFT on medicine management. As part of this, he attends vehicle equipment working groups, the Medicines Governance Group and the monthly Enhanced and Critical Care Group where clinical matters are covered. He also attends all clinical meetings on a national level, conducts staff appraisals and generally takes care of most operational aspects of what goes on at base level.

As the longest-serving member of the DSAA team, Paul has seen a number of changes over the years. He joined the ambulance service in 2000 as a direct entry ambulance technician, becoming a paramedic in 2002. He joined DSAA in 2004, where he worked a one-week-in-four rotation on the helicopter, spending the other three weeks on the road.

'In those days the helicopter was really just a faster route to get people to hospital,' says Paul. 'Paramedics didn't have many additional skills to their colleagues on the road or bring anything like today's enhanced or critical care. Those skills have evolved as the years have passed.' Major trauma centres didn't exist then, so patients would usually be taken to the nearest hospital for further treatment.

The Bölkow 105 (BO 105) helicopter used in the early days was much smaller than the aircraft of today. The paramedic-only crew were very cramped and movement was restricted, as they had to sit sideways with virtually no legroom. Patients were loaded through the tail with monitoring equipment fed through the tunnel with them, from the rear. 'It took longer for the aircraft to start up in those days so you would often be loading patients with the rotors running,' says Paul. 'The noise was incredible. You could barely talk to each other when you didn't have headsets on, you would have to gesture and usher people in and out. If you were on a beach or at a road traffic accident where lots of things were going on, you felt it might be easy to accidently walk into the tail rotor. It was quite scary, noisy, not great for patients – and it brought little more than getting them to hospital quicker than they would by road.'

The service started in a small hangar at Henstridge and the BO 105 shared its space with a host of other small aircraft, including microlights strapped to the ceiling. Once the state-of-the-art EC135 helicopter arrived in 2007, the hangar was no longer deemed secure so the service relocated for just over a year to Westlands in Yeovil before moving back to a purpose-built hangar at Henstridge,

RIGHT **Paul Owen, DSAA Operational Lead and longest-serving crew member.**

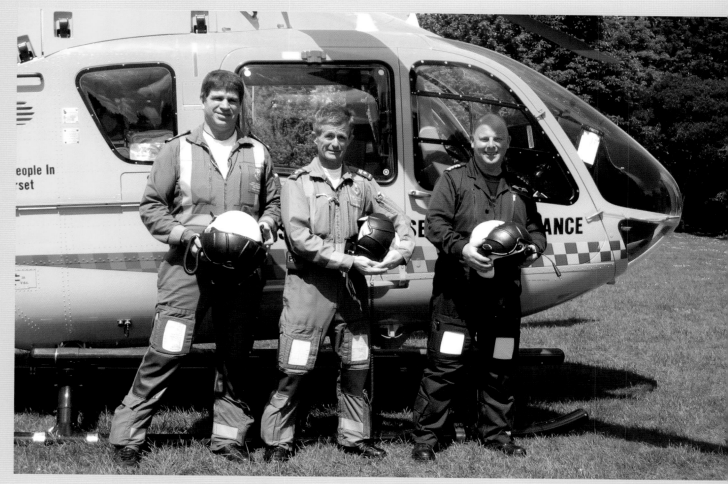

provided by airfield owner Geoff Jarvis, who is a strong supporter of the charity.

Paul became DSAA's clinical support officer in 2007 and staffing changed from a rotational manning system to a more dedicated crew, which was the basis of a structure where people could develop their skills. Paramedics were given the opportunity to perform more complicated procedures and offer patients more options for pain relief. The service developed further when Dr Farhad Islam (Izzy) joined from London HEMS and introduced doctors to the team. Nurses are also part of the mix now and the Critical Care Practitioners come from either paramedic or nursing backgrounds.

Over the past 15 years, Paul has seen a step change. 'Now you have a hospital arriving at the patient's side,' he says. 'We have blood ready to go, one-to-one consultant care, the whole package focused right on the patient. We have gone from a rotational group of paramedics five days a week, to full-time doctor and Critical

Care Cractitioners working 19 hours a day, seven days a week. We can get patients where they really need to go, fully sedated, having received the care while on the aircraft that would previously have been delivered by the hospital.'

Historically, DSAA looked for competent, skilled paramedics. Now they also need to demonstrate more academic ability and be able to follow the master's education pathway. 'We have built time into the rota for hospital rotations and time to work in the community,' says Paul. 'We have the flexibility to use time as we think appropriate to develop our skillsets.'

While the ambulance service was initially somewhat apprehensive about the idea of an air ambulance in Dorset and Somerset, Paul believes the two services have learned much from each other: 'As DSAA moves forward, under the structure and governance of the ambulance service, it benefits them, it benefits us and most of all, it benefits the patients,' he says.

ABOVE Paul Owen (left) with pilots Greg Peacock and Max Hoskins in 2007.

sub-specialty. In April 2016, DSAA made the transition to providing a full critical care service (consisting of at least one Critical Care Practitioner and one critical care doctor for each mission). At the time, this advanced level of care was not widely recognised by many healthcare professionals, meaning that many patients

MEDICAL LEAD: PHIL HYDE

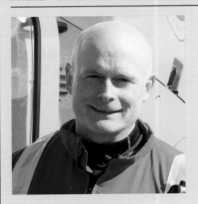

ABOVE Phil Hyde, **DSAA Medical Lead.**

Phil Hyde has worked with DSAA since April 2013, becoming Medical Llead in January 2015. As well as developing the service's critical care model, he has also guided DSAA's extensive clinical governance and multi-professional training and development programme. Actively involved in pre-hospital care since 2003, Phil has volunteered his time to the national development of the sub-specialty of pre-hospital emergency medicine (PHEM); serving as curriculum chair and then assessment chair for the Intercollegiate Board for Training in Pre-Hospital Emergency Medicine (IBTPHEM). Phil also works as a consultant paediatric intensivist at Southampton Children's Hospital and led the development of their major trauma service.

Phil is clear that when utilising public money, DSAA must keep the patient and their best interests at the centre of all decisions. 'It's essential that we utilise the money raised by the public in the most efficient and just fashion for the benefit of the local population,' says Phil. 'We collect data about patient need and the care provided to patients; we then utilise these data to systematically improve the service for the population; this is achieved within the NHS governance frameworks.'

Accurate and complete data about patient care is essential to provide evidence for future developments in patient treatments. To enable this, DSAA supported Dr Mike Eddie to create a relational database called 'PHEMnet'. Phil sees the potential of the PHEMnet data system to enable improved care for patients across the UK as an exciting example of air ambulance-led innovation.

Phil believes that advocacy for critically injured and ill patients is about more than the medical care they receive. 'Air ambulances are extremely well placed to inform, support and lead the prevention of injury and illness. The unique, humbling and privileged exposure that air ambulance teams have to the life journeys of patients and their families can be utilised to reduce the burden of disease within the community.'

faced with a life-threatening illness or injury were possibly not getting the care they might need.

Even today, air ambulance services don't always have doctors on board. Having chosen to move to the critical care model, DSAA is one of the few air ambulance services with a critical care team operating day and night, using consultant-level doctors, enabling the teams to respond flexibly to patients' needs. While the master's qualification obtained by DSAA practitioners means that the practical roles of practitioner and doctor are interchangeable now, when it comes to governance and overall responsibility for the patient, the final responsibility rests with the doctor. In some parts of the country, there simply aren't enough doctors at this level to join local air ambulance crews, but it's also important to get the staffing balance right: having too many team members can cause just as many problems as having too few, as individuals won't get enough exposure to real cases and their skills may fade or stagnate.

'There are many models out there,' explains Bill. 'Doctor-led, doctor-enabled and so on. We decided on a very flat-structured model, where the critical care team has one doctor and one – or in some cases two – practitioners, depending on whether we are day or night flying. But they are in effect operator one and operator two; no one is the leader, it's a team effort. That has permeated everything that we do.'

While the twin-paramedic model had enabled DSAA to provide fast and effective care for its patients, the critical care model allowed it to deliver an enhanced service, administering drugs (including pre-hospital anaesthetics), performing surgical procedures and giving organ support to critically ill patients at the scene of an incident, on any given day.

DSAA has established its own clinical governance approach, which sits comfortably within the SWASFT NHS clinical governance system. It consists of regular case reviews and a formal review each month of its clinical administration, which looks at the care provided to patients, learning points for the whole team, changes to the system to design out error, training of staff, and the management of drugs and equipment. This all helps to build a knowledge-based, learning organisation.

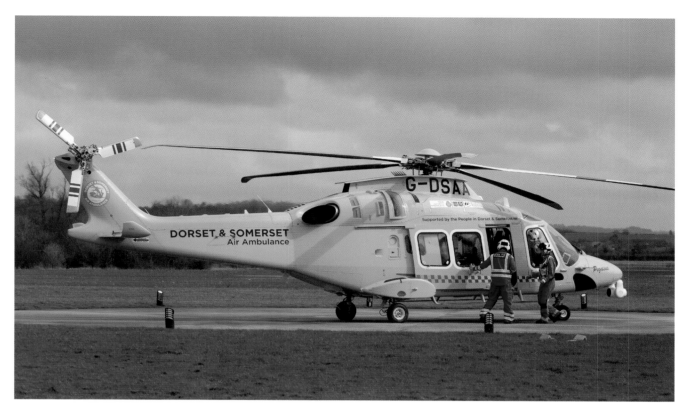

The clinical team structure and ethos is now well established and lessons have been pulled through into the rest of the charity. The trustees, charity staff and volunteers now have much more interaction with clinical crew and former patients, which gives them a greater sense of purpose and of being part of one team.

ABOVE AND BELOW LEFT The Critical Care model, coupled with the flexibility and cabin space of the AW169, allows DSAA to deliver an enhanced service.

BELOW While the roles of practitioner and doctor are virtually interchangeable, when it comes to governance and overall responsibility for the patient, the final responsibility rests with the doctor.

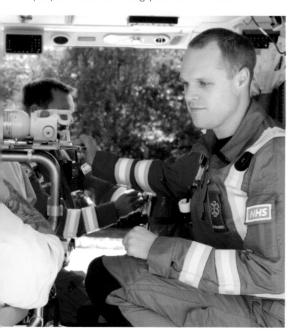

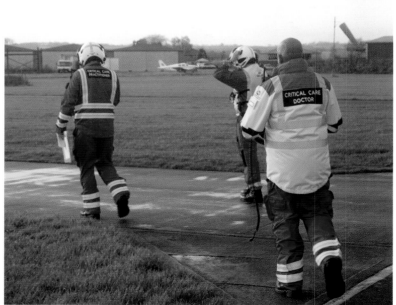

Matt Sawyer is one of a new cohort of trainees who have joined DSAA. Matt qualified as a paramedic in 2008 and in 2018 he started working part-time as an Advanced Clinical Practitioner (ACP) in emergency care and as a trainee Critical Care Practitioner (CCP) for DSAA. He has been with DSAA for six months and his schedule is split between his hospital job in the emergency department and the air ambulance.

Competition to work on the air ambulance is fierce. There were four full-time equivalent positions when Matt was recruited and some 120 people applied. To get onto the selection programme, candidates needed to demonstrate that they meet certain essential and desirable criteria, such as a proven track record for academic or career progression, and robust clinical and communication skills. A written exam followed, testing his background knowledge of the anatomy, physiology,

pharmacology, operational and clinical practice of pre-hospital medicine. They also had to run through a number of scenarios that tested their clinical, technical and non-technical skills, as well as demonstrate a good basic knowledge of how an air ambulance and critical care team operates. Finally, candidates had to give a presentation to a panel of senior clinicians and executives from the charity, followed by an interview.

Matt's experience as an ACP has given him a solid foundation for his role at the air ambulance. ACPs are clinicians that come from a non-medical background but who practise with a high degree of independence, beyond their traditional professional boundary. ACPs are responsible for assessing patients and making decisions about their care. In an emergency care environment, ACPs are typically nurses or paramedics, but sometimes physiotherapists or other healthcare practitioners.

'ACPs are trained to work in all areas of the emergency department, to assess and treat patients right across the spectrum from minor injuries or illness to life-threatening problems,' explains Matt. 'We work closely with medical colleagues and have a role in education, quality improvement and leadership within the department.'

While it's generally accepted that an ACP has a similar scope of practice to a mid-level A&E doctor, of course there are things a doctor can do that an ACP cannot. On the flip side, ACPs often have skills or experience that a doctor doesn't necessarily possess and unlike doctors in postgraduate training, ACPs don't usually rotate to different roles or hospitals so represent a stable workforce. 'Because of our background as allied health professionals, we often spend more time with patients and perform basic care alongside more complex interventions,' says Matt. 'We've often also got other little tricks that are of benefit, such as being able to package/unpackage patients smoothly, keep them comfortable on trolleys or help them off the floor.'

Matt started his role at DSAA in a supernumerary capacity, undertaking training at the airbase with the other doctors and CCPs.

BELOW Matt Sawyer, DSAA trainee Critical Care Practitioner.

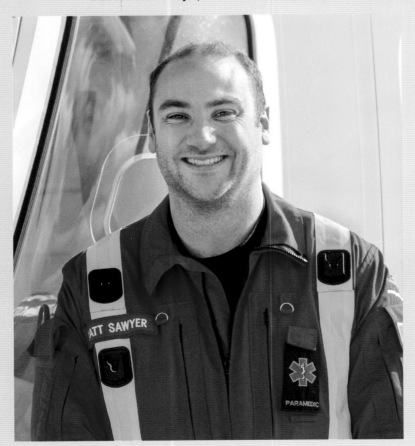

Among other things, this involved using all the equipment and learning how each piece works, when it is needed and how to troubleshoot any problems that arise with using it. He built on this with lots of simulation-based training, before he and the rest of the trainees started going out on the helicopter or rapid response vehicle as additional crew members. This gave them invaluable exposure and insight into what they needed to do as part of the clinical team and as the aviation Technical Crew Member (TCM), while still working in a way that didn't compromise any patient care.

'Every single day we train as a team,' says Matt. 'The duty team will identify their educational needs from an aviation and clinical perspective and throughout the day, when they're not on a job, will undertake practical and theoretical training in those areas.'

Trainees start by accompanying the duty team on missions during the day, but they must gain experience in doing the job before they can go out on night missions. They first have to pass an assessment, running through a scenario where their ability to troubleshoot different problems and ability to make safe decisions are tested against set criteria. In the early months of working for DSAA, all trainees take the TCM course (see page 141), which provides the additional aviation training to become a TCM. This includes mission planning and navigation skills, aircraft safety and an exam, written by SAS, based on European Aviation Safety Agency (EASA) guidance on what a TCM should be able to do. After a consolidation period of several months the trainees undertake further training and assessment to ensure they can perform as a night TCM. This includes use of Night Vision Goggles (NVGs), operation of the Trakkabeam and other aviation and human factors related to operating HEMS aircraft at night.

Trainees also take part in the monthly training session that takes place on the base for all the crew. This always has a different theme: recently all team members have undertaken an annual assessment of their competence to conduct surgical procedures out of hospital, such as a surgical airway

or perform an amputation, thoracotomy (opening a patient's chest to gain access to the heart), or a resuscitative hysterotomy (an emergency caesarean when the mother may die immediately). Some months the training is very practical, using lots of equipment or doing simulations on major incidents or extricating people from cars. Other sessions are more theoretical, with lectures delivered on different issues, such as human physiology or pharmacology.

There isn't really a set amount of time in which a trainee qualifies – previous trainees have taken anything from a year to 18 months. 'We all have different experience and knowledge underpinning our skills and learn at different rates,' says Matt. 'But there are some things that have to be done in real life before the training is complete, and it is a matter of chance as to when it happens.'

Regular reviews take place and each trainee is assigned a mentor or two, who take a special interest in their development and support them along the way. Any of the qualified CCPs and established doctors can contribute to a trainee's development by signing off competencies as they go along, and verifying that the trainee has done certain things in practice, such as perform a pre-hospital emergency anaesthetic. Final sign-off happens with Paul Owen and Phil Hyde, who review a trainee's portfolio and ensure it meets the required standard.

Matt is finding that both his roles have a huge crossover, with a knowledge and skill mix that really benefits him in both settings. He has picked up a lot of experience from the emergency department that helps him deliver effective pre-hospital critical care, while his training with DSAA has added value to how he works in the emergency department too.

'There are only a few non-medical practitioners nationally following this pathway as a clinician working across both these environments,' says Matt. 'So I feel very privileged to be doing it and helping patients both in and out of hospital, and to be helping shape a multi-professional pathway to develop other clinicians.'

Claire applied to the ambulance service in 2005 and joined as a direct entry ambulance technician in 2006. In 2009, she qualified as a paramedic through the Institute of Health and Care Development. At the beginning of Claire's career, Ken Wenman, chief executive of SWASFT, had explained to her that the paramedic role would diversify and develop over the coming years and the critical care model was one that always interested her. Claire undertook a number of extra courses to further her education and her continuing professional development (CPD), before joining DSAA as a HEMS paramedic in 2012. This was before the Critical Care model had been realised, and when the service was staffed by HEMS paramedics with extended skills, focusing more on accessing the patient quickly and rapid transportation to hospital.

In 2013, DSAA's resident consultant, Dr Farhad Islam, developed an award-winning educational programme in conjunction with the University of Hertfordshire, which enabled the paramedics to complete their training as Critical Care Paramedics. To facilitate this, a team of doctors began flying with the paramedics over the following years, and DSAA became a full-time critical care team in 2016. 'This greatly enhanced the level of care we could offer patients at the roadside, but also supported and hugely developed the practice of the Critical Care Practitioners,' says Claire.

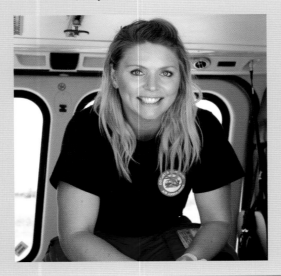

RIGHT Claire Baker, DSAA Critical Care Practitioner.

Claire has continued on her academic path while at DSAA and has recently completed her master's degree in advanced paramedic practice (critical care). The course was fully funded by the charity. 'From a personal point of view, coming out the other side of a master's and feeling fully developed in professional terms is far more than I could have ever imagined seven years ago,' she says. 'Working with a select few consultants in anaesthetics and emergency medicine has been an amazing opportunity and one that wouldn't have been available if I wasn't on the air ambulance. The learning that takes place through osmosis has really helped consolidate my academic work.'

Her time with DSAA has been quite different to her time with the ambulance service. 'As a HEMS paramedic, I see a totally different type of patient,' she says. 'We are strategically deployed to care for the most critically unwell patients in the region.' Along with her DSAA colleagues, Claire is experienced in treating patients suffering severe trauma and acute medical illnesses, as well as dealing with patients and bystanders who are witnessing it. 'Because you see high numbers of these incidents you become somewhat acclimatised to them,' she explains. 'Colleagues are relieved that we can come along and help them with patients that are more difficult to manage. Repeated exposure and experience with these sort of cases make us more practised at dealing with them, both clinically and emotionally.'

Being funded by the charity, as opposed to the NHS, DSAA also has the opportunity to create a different clinical environment for its patients and can develop its practice and equipment to fit.

'We have the luxury of time and money that no other part of the NHS has,' says Claire. 'It's taken a long time to get to this point, but through careful development of the service and working closely with the charity, we are lucky enough to have these opportunities to push the boundaries of pre-hospital care for the patient.'

Key partnerships

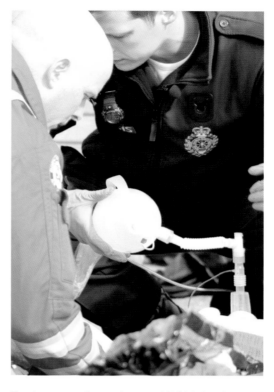

As might be expected, DSAA works in close partnership with the NHS on a number of levels. Its main NHS partner organisation is the South Western Ambulance Service NHS Foundation Trust (SWASFT). SWASFT covers the largest geographic area of any ambulance service in the country and has five air ambulance charities operating within its area.

Supporting SWASFT colleagues is an essential part of DSAA's role. 'There are some 2,000 ambulance service staff employed by SWASFT,' says Phil Hyde. 'Those 2,000 pairs of eyes on the ground create an incredible surveillance system of people looking for critically ill and injured patients, which we want to access. As the ambulance service's critical care asset, we want to support them as much as possible, breaking down any historical barriers to working together, particularly if they are trying to cope with patients that we could help them with.'

While some other air ambulances employ their doctors directly, and some are fully funded by the NHS, DSAA's view is that it is in the best interests of its patients to have a close relationship with the hospitals. All DSAA doctors are employed by NHS Acute Hospital Trusts across the region, and DSAA funds the doctors' time through service level agreements (SLAs), with the doctors' employing NHS Trust. This approach was felt by DSAA to fit most comfortably with its team ethos. Having ties with the hospitals that extend beyond the

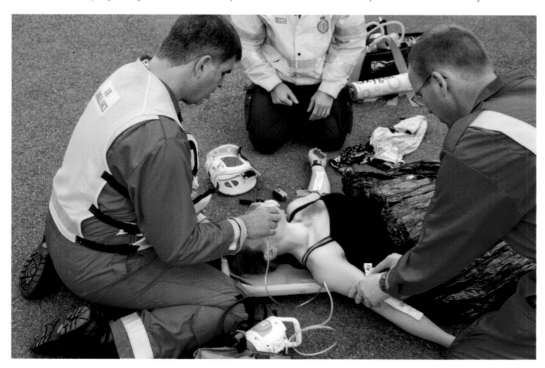

emergency department door creates more trust between organisations and clinicians and it is felt that patients enjoy a smoother transition from the pre-hospital to the in-hospital environment as a result.

DSAA's first formal partnership with a local Acute Trust was established with Royal Bournemouth General Hospital and now includes Yeovil District Hospital, Musgrove Park Hospital in Taunton, Poole General Hospital, Dorset County Hospital in Dorchester, Royal United Hospital Bath, University Hospital Southampton and even Hereford County Hospital, giving a full spread across the South West of England.

This close working partnership with the NHS is not necessarily the model for all air ambulances in the UK. Others, for various reasons, have chosen a different course. Some, like London's Air Ambulance, work within the NHS, while others operate in a more distanced way, where the only link with the NHS is the phone call that tasks them. Air ambulance services in the UK operate very differently: geographies are different, demographics are different and significantly, the way in which the NHS itself operates in different regions is so varied. Each regional air ambulance has to fit in with local requirements. Although air ambulances often refer to patients as 'theirs', they are in fact under the umbrella of the NHS Ambulance Service, which has the statutory authority. That is why the air ambulance must be tasked by the ambulance service to undertake HEMS.

HEMS desk

In 2007, SWASFT created a permanent Helicopter Emergency Medical Service (HEMS) desk to cover the South West region and recruited three dispatchers to work on what was then the first full-time HEMS desk in the country. The desk is paid for by the five air ambulance charities that it serves (Dorset and Somerset Air Ambulance, Devon Air Ambulance, Cornwall Air Ambulance, Great Western Air Ambulance Charity and Wiltshire Air Ambulance) and the charities work closely to ensure that mutual aid is provided and that boundaries do not affect a patient's care. Once the 999 call comes in, regardless of who or where a patient is, the most appropriate asset (which is not always a helicopter) will be dispatched.

Located at one of the SWASFT clinical hubs in Exeter, the desk is staffed by a team of eight HEMS dispatchers, who cover the desk for a 20-hour period while any of the air ambulances are operational. The team is responsible for deploying all six air ambulance helicopters (Devon Air Ambulance has two aircraft) across the South West region. This is a dynamic and vast geographical area and, should the need arise, the team can also call on support from HM Coastguard, the police and search and rescue.

Before the decision is taken to deploy an air ambulance, a number of factors have to be considered. There are six criteria that dictate whether or not the helicopter will be automatically dispatched. If a patient has been run over by a car, fallen from a height of more than three storeys, or received a stab or

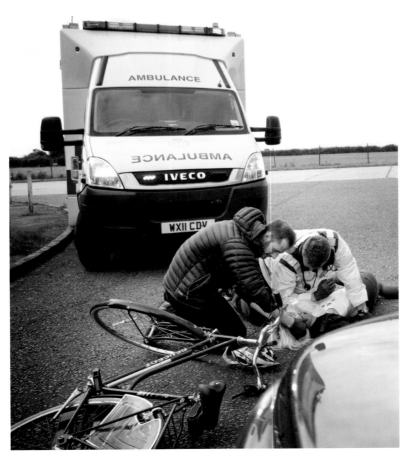

BELOW DSAA enjoys a close working partnership with the NHS. *(Simon Pryor)*

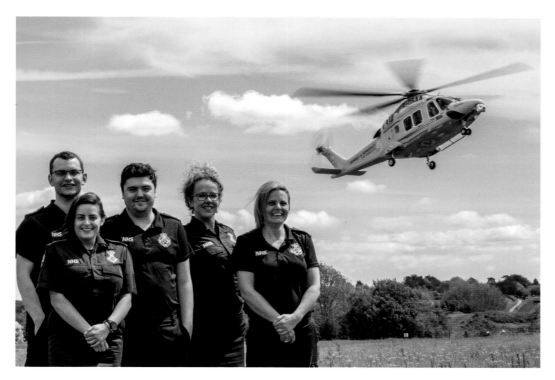

gunshot wound to the torso, the air ambulance will be tasked. It will also be dispatched if the patient has been ejected from a vehicle during a road traffic accident, if they are in the car with a passenger or driver who has died, or if they have fallen under or been struck by a train. 'Under these circumstances we would dispatch an air ambulance even if the job was right next to a hospital,' explains Paul Holmes, HEMS Dispatch Control Officer, 'as our clinicians have the necessary skills to assist.'

The dispatchers have a number of screens that help them monitor every 999 call made to the control room. Every single 999 call is triaged and if an emergency call comes in but the description doesn't meet one of the HEMS desk's automatic dispatch criteria, they will listen in to the call in order to assess the situation. Land ambulances are automatically sent out (by land dispatchers) to calls that have been triaged as an emergency response and tasking an air ambulance to a job does not have any impact on this. Despite the specialist skills and rapid response that an air ambulance can provide, it may still be faster or more appropriate to take the patient on to hospital afterwards by land.

When a job is identified, the HEMS desk calls the respective air ambulance crew and gives them key information, such as the location and grid reference, so the route can be planned straight away. The HEMS mapping system shows the position of all the land ambulances, air ambulances, community first responders, doctors and rapid response vehicles, and helps the dispatcher identify the location of the incident, appraise the landing conditions and

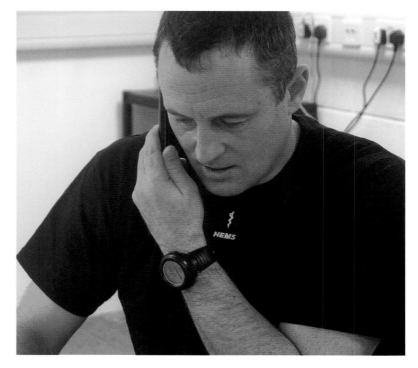

give the air ambulance crew an idea of how close they may be able to land. The dispatcher then updates the crews in the air and on land as the situation unfolds, letting them know the status of the patient, respective times of arrival and if circumstances change and one of them can stand down.

The HEMS desk also sends daily tasking sheets to each of the air ambulance charities, as well as monthly reports. Everything that happens on the desk is logged – whether an aircraft attends the scene of an incident or whether it can't go to a job because it is already committed or offline for some reason. This data provides an overview of the activity of all air ambulances within SWASFT. Before the advent of night flying, the HEMS desk would do out-of-hours searches for HEMS data, to assess which of the jobs that came in overnight would have had a helicopter tasked to it. The results of this data formed part of the case for extending flying hours.

Each dispatcher undergoes specialist training, both in the classroom and with an experienced HEMS dispatcher, before taking up the role. During the week of classroom training, the dispatcher learns about aviation safety, weather restrictions and air traffic control rules, so they are aware of the problems that an air ambulance might face in certain situations.

Further training days take place throughout the year, including visits to the airbases to meet the crews or attend governance meetings. These help dispatchers stay abreast of safety issues and keep up to date with the clinical skills offered by each of the air ambulance services, as well as anything else that may be changing with the crews or aircraft. Flying days are also held, where dispatchers go out in the aircraft to observe what the aircrew does and see first-hand some of the issues the helicopter faces, such as landing in tight spots. This gives dispatchers a thorough idea of what goes on while in the air and can help to explain some of the questions that they might be asked by the crew during a call, or why the pilot may turn off the radio if he is trying to focus on landing. These contact days also strengthen the bond between all the teams.

'It is a role that is very challenging but also very rewarding,' says Paul. 'Every day you are at work, you never know what is going to happen next, but you always go home feeling like you have made a difference.'

Carriage of blood components

When patients suffer life-threatening bleeding caused by major trauma or acute medical conditions, emergency blood transfusions are usually given. An estimated 40% of trauma deaths are due to bleeding, so being able to carry and administer blood components to these patients before they get to hospital can be a matter of life or death. Blood components are packed red cells, plasma, platelets or cryoprecipitate. DSAA currently uses packed red cells and thawed plasma.

In June 2016, DSAA announced a collaboration with Dorset County Hospital, Devon Freewheelers, SWASFT and the Henry Surtees Foundation, which resulted in patients being able to receive blood components at the scene of an incident. Following months of research, the charity's critical care team worked extremely hard on identifying the best way to deliver, implement and fund the project.

In a bid to ensure that patients have enough blood to keep them alive until they reach hospital, DSAA now carries four units of O-type red blood cells, as well as plasma. It is one of four air ambulance charities in the UK to carry a combination of blood and plasma.

Advice from the military suggests that if a patient is bleeding to death, they should receive both packed red cells (which carry oxygen) and plasma (which carries the clotting factors to help stop the bleeding). Freeze-dried plasma was initially selected as the preferred option to fresh frozen plasma as it has a shelf-life of approximately 18 months and can be made up when needed – unlike fresh frozen plasma, which has a five-day shelf-life after being thawed. However, a worldwide shortage of freeze-dried plasma has prompted DSAA to adopt fresh frozen plasma. Because of the shelf-life issue, this is clearly a much more expensive option. However, DSAA now has a system that places the thawed plasma with

DEVON FREEWHEELERS

Devon Freewheelers is a volunteer-based charity that provides an out-of-hours service to the NHS. Using marked blood bikes and cars, it transports urgently needed blood and medical supplies between hospitals. Besides the charity's core work, the volunteers also transport medical equipment, surgical equipment, medication, donor breast milk, patient notes and, more recently, blood, tissue and organs for transplant. The riders and drivers are volunteers who give up their free time to help provide this life-saving service.

Since DSAA began carrying blood products in 2016, Devon Freewheelers have ensured that blood is delivered to the clinical care team every 48 hours. Each driver is on call for two days, enabling them to complete the scheduled resupply and exchange of blood on one day and be available to respond to any unscheduled resupply if it is used. The driver collects the blood from the Dorchester County Hospital blood bank and transports it to DSAA's Henstridge airbase. There they will exchange it with either the unused blood products, or in the case of an unscheduled run, the used product container. They will then return the blood transit containers back to the blood bank at the hospital.

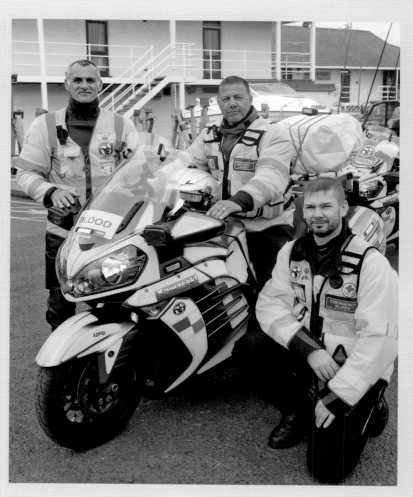

ABOVE AND BELOW Volunteers from the Devon Freewheelers deliver the blood and fresh frozen plasma to DSAA.

BELOW Martin Warden, a member of the Devon Freewheelers team.

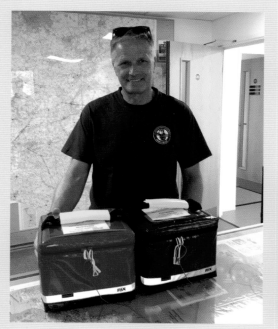

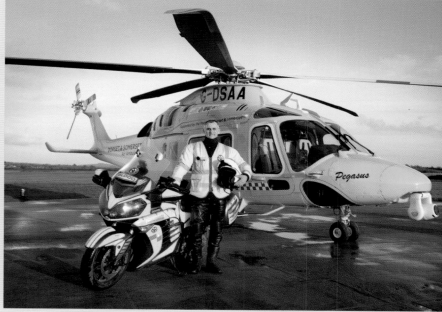

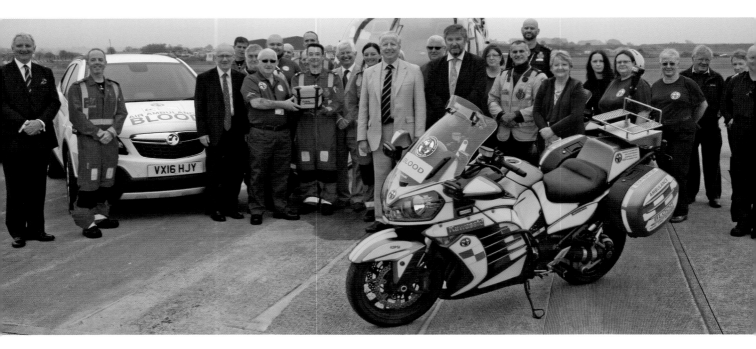

ABOVE An estimated 40% of trauma deaths are due to bleeding, so being able to carry and administer blood components to these patients before they get to hospital can be a matter of life or death.

the service for two days of its five-day lifespan before being returned to the hospital for use, and DSAA shares the cost accordingly.

Developing the blood service is expensive, and DSAA was grateful to receive significant financial assistance from the Henry Surtees Foundation, which covered both the set-up costs of the service and the leasing costs of the Vauxhall Mokka 4x4 driven by the Devon Freewheelers, the charity that delivers the blood to DSAA.

Specialist hospital equipment is required to pre-condition the blood, as is careful transportation to and from hospital to the airbase and a dedicated, safe storage place. Special equipment is also required to keep the blood cold on the aircraft and also to warm it while it is being transfused to the patient. The blood is stored in temperature-regulated 'golden hour' boxes, which keep the blood under 6°C (43°F) for up to 72 hours. These boxes require conditioning in order to function (a process of freezing and partial thawing) using -40°C (also -40°F) freezers provided specifically for this purpose. In order to withstand carriage on the helicopter, the boxes are packed and

sealed prior to dispatch by the Dorset County Hospital Transfusion Team and contain a temperature logging device that ensures the blood temperature is monitored while it is out of the hospital environment.

Volunteers from the Devon Freewheelers deliver the blood and fresh frozen plasma to DSAA on blood bikes and in a sponsored car. If the 'golden hour' box is unopened at the end of the 48-hour period, it will be collected by the Devon Freewheelers and returned to the hospital, where it will be reissued and utilised. Similarly, if blood is used during a shift, the HEMS desk contacts the hospital's Transfusion Laboratory and the Devon Freewheelers deliver additional stocks within a matter of hours.

In July 2018, DSAA started carrying 'shock packs', which contain four units of blood and four units of thawed plasma in its liquid form. Having these products immediately at hand means that the team has an amazing resource with which to resuscitate both adults and children who are suffering from severe trauma, or other conditions in which very large quantities of blood have been lost.

While, to the layperson, the decision to carry blood in the air ambulance seems very straightforward, in reality, it takes an enormous amount of careful consideration and detailed planning by a number of organisations to make it happen.

CRITICAL CARE PRACTITIONER: MICHELLE WALKER

Before the provision of blood components could commence, the critical care team needed to spend a number of months researching how best to deliver and implement the project, which was challenging given the little research in this area that was available at the time. Critical Care Practitioner Michelle Walker and Intensive Care Consultant Ian Mew were instrumental in carrying out this work.

Michelle joined the ambulance service in 2003 and moved to DSAA in 2012. 'When I started out we only had doctors flying with us once a week,' says Michelle. 'I used to feel really frustrated when we had a patient who needed blood and we couldn't provide it.' She and her colleagues saw a number of patients die who they firmly believed would have had a better chance of survival had they received blood at the scene, but there was little or no evidence to suggest this was the case.

Ian has strong links with Dorset County Hospital, so they started there, looking at the governance structure, the logistics of transporting the blood, storing it at the right temperatures, warming it up before administering to a patient and the special equipment involved, such as the types of bag in which they could keep the blood components, all to comply with legal requirements.

Now that the process is established, part of Michelle's role is to do a monthly audit on the units of blood, making sure each unit is accounted for and recording which patient received it. Where possible, she follows up on patients, cross-checking paperwork with the records held by hospitals and SWASFT. DSAA clinicians use an anonymised database for recording all incidents that occur during a mission, including the delivery of blood.

Michelle is also responsible for updating the Standard Operating Procedures and assisting with annual training days that simulate surgical procedures and administering blood components, using medical meat products, which allow for more realistic and robust training. Medical meat comes from approved providers, which adhere to strict conditions.

As part of her master's degree, Michelle studied the data and, although the numbers were initially small (only 50 to 60 patients each year have been unwell enough to receive blood products), after 18 months' worth of data she could see that patients who would previously have died on the scene are getting to hospital.

'I can't say for sure yet that we have saved X amount of people by administering blood products,' says Michelle. 'But collecting the data should enable a retrospective study. So far, the evidence suggests it is making a difference and among us, as clinicians treating these very critically unwell patients, we definitely wouldn't want to be without it.'

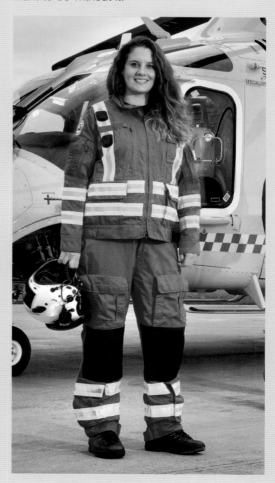

LEFT Michelle Walker, DSAA Critical Care Practitioner.

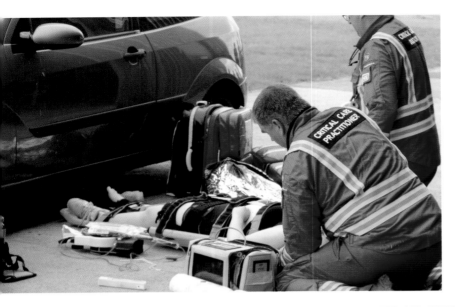

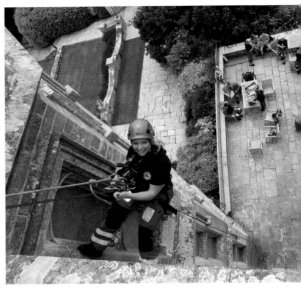

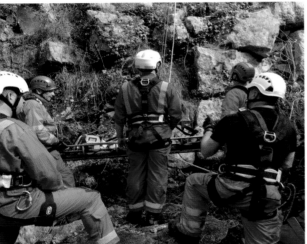

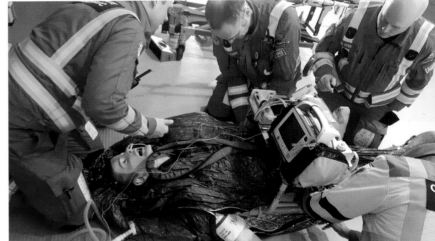

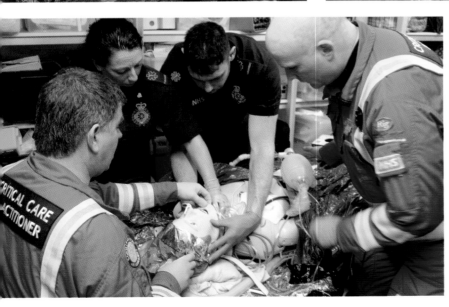

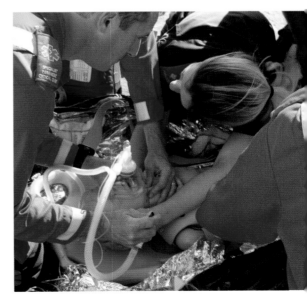

Training

Every month, the whole DSAA team trains together to ensure that the highest quality of care is provided to patients. Training is led by Team Education Facilitator Emily Cooper and Critical Care Practitioner Owen Hammett. These monthly sessions are based on the pre-hospital emergency medicine (PHEM) curriculum used by the Faculty of Pre-hospital Care and covers working in emergency medical systems, providing pre-hospital emergency medical care, using pre-hospital equipment, supporting rescue and extrication, supporting safe patient transfer, supporting emergency preparedness and response, operational practice, team resource management and clinical governance. The monthly training supports the DSAA team in managing medically ill and traumatically injured patients of all ages (newborns, children and adults).

The training team set out the content they want to cover each month, then sit down and work out what simulations would be beneficial, where there might be particular learning requirements that need addressing, or whether team members have been faced with a particularly challenging situation and want to demonstrate to their colleagues how they have handled it and discuss how this could be managed in the future.

All the simulations are designed to draw focus to a particular challenging aspect or medical condition that the team may come across during a tasking. After each simulated scenario the team debriefs and discusses them in detail, looking particularly at any critical decision-making points. The simulation is sometimes repeated, implementing any changes, with the purpose of then making those improvements at the roadside.

One scenario covered a patient with a penetrating chest wound, who had gone into cardiac arrest. In real life, the team would be expected to open the chest to find the source of bleeding and repair it. In the training scenario, they used a manikin's head and medical meat products, enabling team members to put knife to skin, open the chest, gain access to the heart and repair the injury to the ventricle.

The team has access to a written-off car,

as well as an old aircraft fuselage that they can use for a range of patient simulations and extrications. Most training sessions involve the use of infant, child and adult manikins, all of which have been purchased by the charity. One very high-tech manikin can be plugged into a laptop and programmed to do particular things, such as cough, blink, talk and have an elevated heart rate, while the less high-tech manikins often find themselves thrown into bushes or under the car. The team also uses actors who come in and are given a list of symptoms to perform. 'When the crew practise on a real person it really increases the fidelity,' says Emily. 'They have to talk to someone, hold their hand, reassure them, while also treating and managing their emergency medical condition.'

OPPOSITE Training takes place every month and the team undertakes simulations covering a wide variety of scenarios.

BELOW Emily Cooper, DSAA team education facilitator.

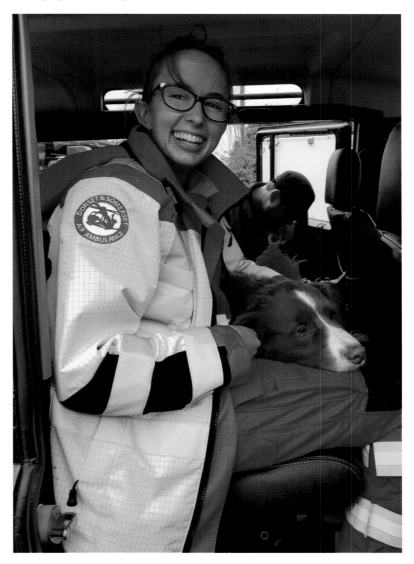

CRITICAL CARE PRACTITIONER: OWEN HAMMETT

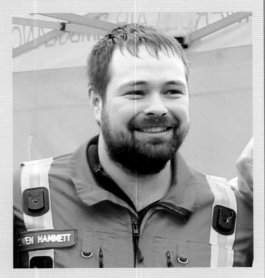

RIGHT Owen Hammett, DSAA Critical Care Practitioner.

Owen is a registered nurse by training. His father was a paramedic and that instilled in Owen an interest in pre-hospital care. Once he had qualified as a nurse, Owen moved into emergency medicine in a major trauma centre and gained experience looking after extremely sick patients. He then moved to a specialist technological and transfer role in an intensive care unit (ICU), specialising in specific life-support equipment, from ventilators to filters; and in moving ICU patients around the hospital, for example to the MRI scanner. He was also part of the paediatric intensive care retrieval service for a regional cardiac centre, collecting children from local hospitals and bringing them to the most suitable hospital by land or air.

Owen joined DSAA in 2017 and leads the training programme with colleague Emily Cooper. His specific experience with life-support equipment was part of the reason that he was selected to be one of the clinicians to liaise with Specialist Aviation Services on the medical refit of the AW169.

'It doesn't matter whether you are a paramedic or a nurse, the care we deliver to patients is exactly the same,' he says. 'We just have different backgrounds, but these differences are healthy as the crew members can learn a lot from each other.'

Emily is responsible for the scenario writing, timetabling and facilitation on the day, but each month a doctor and Critical Care Practitioner are allocated to support her and contribute their ideas. Depending on the subject matter, DSAA will often also draw upon a pool of experts to come in and share their experience and knowledge with the crew.

DSAA also holds inter-professional training days involving other agencies, including the police, RNLI, HM Coastguard and fire and rescue. One particular training exercise involved more than 100 people in a large-scale search and rescue simulation. 'The programme is very varied,' says Emily. 'We push the limits on training – we have even been down old bomb shelters to run simulations in small spaces. We come up with ideas and scenarios and then put out feelers to see if anyone is able to support us. Usually we get a very positive response.'

Each year the pilots hold a day dedicated to aviation training, where they put on a range of activities, such as providing updates on the performance of the aircraft or looking at improving and building on crew resource management. The entire DSAA team also undertakes a team-building day every year.

The training programme continually improves the team's dynamics and performance. Its ethos is simple: DSAA's crew trains how they perform. 'We go out in the cold and rain, in the wet and mud, because that is where patients are,' explains Emily. 'We don't just sit in the classroom and talk.'

Outreach

The emergency services sector contains a vast mix of different skills and disciplines, from control centre dispatchers and community first responders (CFRs), to experienced pre-hospital emergency medicine (PHEM) doctors working with the UK's air ambulances and ambulance service crews, fire and rescue service personnel, the police, RNLI and the coastguard. To ensure that its patients have the best possible chance of survival, DSAA's critical care team has developed a major outreach initiative to educate and empower emergency service colleagues to mobilise critical care for patients in need.

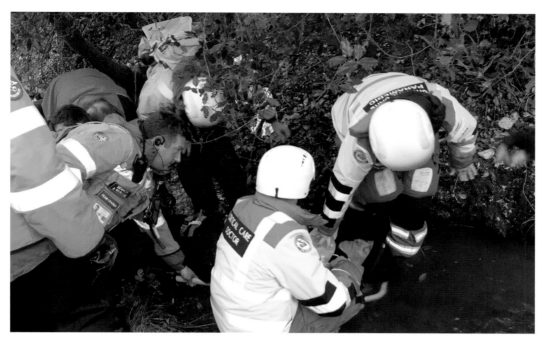

LEFT DSAA's outreach
initiative educates and
empowers emergency
service colleagues to
mobilise critical care
for patients in need.

Collaborative working between emergency
and rescue services, dispatchers, managers,
hospitals and all individuals concerned with
the patient is essential for a scene to work
effectively. Using an open, approachable and
supportive ethos, the outreach programme
gives professionals and students alike an
opportunity to collaborate, reflect, learn and
improve, all for the benefit of patients.

The outreach programme is led by Critical
Care Paramedic Neil Bizzell, who joined
DSAA in 2015. In the early days, Neil felt
there was often a lack of understanding on
everyone's parts at the scene of an incident:
road ambulance crews were removed from
the air crews, people didn't know each other
by name and they only came into contact with
each other in a dynamic, potentially stressful
scene. Despite this, everyone was able to work
together professionally, but it was sometimes a
challenge for the different people attending the
scene to communicate effectively.

Neil's starting point was to go back to the
very beginning, before an incident takes place,
to see who the DSAA team engaged with
before and during the scene. Firstly, the control
services: without which DSAA wouldn't know
about the patients in the first place. While
trauma calls are relatively straightforward for
the dedicated HEMS desk to identify, DSAA
also needs them to identify appropriate medical

calls. 'We really rely on our clinical supervisors in
the control room, our dispatchers, our 999 call
handlers and the HEMS desk operators to all
have a heightened awareness of our capability
and how we can support them,' explains Neil.
'The earlier we can be dispatched, the quicker
we can arrive to add enhanced critical care to
support the ambulance teams on scene.'

After the call has been made, a number
of potential different groups come together
and have to integrate into a dynamic incident
scene. CFRs dispatched by SWASFT are often
first on the scene after a 999 call. CFRs have
solid basic training and offer assistance where

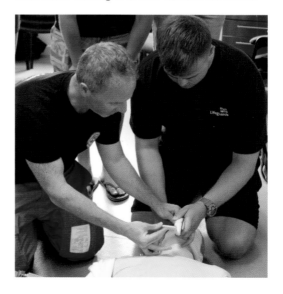

LEFT RNLI Lifeguards
from Weymouth
learning key skills
during an outreach
exercise.

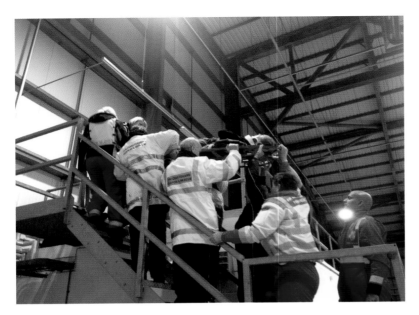

ABOVE **Simulating a cliff rescue with a team from the coastguard.**

possible, waiting with the patient until the ambulance arrives. CFRs are volunteers and can be found in all regions of the UK, especially in rural areas. Regular engagement with CFRs greatly increases their understanding of the air ambulance's capabilities, enabling them to identify potential incidents where DSAA should be deployed.

CFRs are then backed up by an ambulance crew, possibly with a manager, operations officer or learning and development officer present if it's a serious incident. There could also be police, coastguard or RNLI on the scene, or other air ambulances. There may even be a university student in the land ambulance. Students are often young trainee paramedics and for them, this could be their first exposure to patients requiring critical care and at a time in their career when they are impressionable, so it's important that the culture of being 'one team' is demonstrated.

The DSAA team is always learning how to better integrate into a scene. When the air ambulance arrives at an incident, the team likes to have a clinical update, rather than a handover. 'We build upon the clinical interventions and emergency care that has already been given by those attending,' says Neil. 'We may end up transporting the patient away but by no means should anyone feel we have taken over a scene, we are simply there to support the ambulance crews.

'We may all be wearing different colours,'

continues Neil, 'but we are all working towards the same ultimate goal of caring for the patient.' It is essential that if any one of these individuals has any concerns that may manifest later, they all know that DSAA is an open organisation and can always be contacted afterwards to discuss things.

The outreach programme exists not only to forge and improve relations across this emergency services community, but also to inspire those caring for critically ill or critically injured patients to continue to improve their practice, and be given the foundation to pursue a career in pre-hospital critical care medicine. Ultimately, the focus is on saving lives and improving patient pathways.

The DSAA critical care team carries out a number of structured engagement events, which include talks at regional centres, joint training exercises at the Henstridge airbase and in different pre-hospital care environments. Teamwork is key and the programme involves presentations, group discussions, workshops and scenarios that explain and demonstrate the capabilities of DSAA's clinical team. It encourages integration and communication and has forged collaborative working practices with many colleagues in the emergency services. Improved inter-agency co-operation has enabled better decision-making when tasking assets to assist a patient and helps the receiving hospital better prepare for a patient's arrival.

On a more personal level, DSAA also holds 'acquaint days' where the team has informal workshops covering a range of scenarios, with a discussion at the end of the day explaining what the service does and why they do it. These enable DSAA to develop its service, thanks to the experience of its colleagues from elsewhere. 'People know each other's names or at least recognise each other and find it much easier to engage with others when they have a direct relationship with people,' says Neil. During the day, participants often come up with interesting questions or suggestions about what can be done to make the whole process more efficient. One such suggestion was the prompt cards that DSAA use, which have proved really useful. The cards explain to outside colleagues what the critical care team at DSAA can help with, what could be done to facilitate the patient's onward treatment pathways, and how the patient can be packaged.

A range of immersive educational days see the DSAA team engage with many different local organisations, including universities, CFR groups, ambulance service staff, lifeguards, neighbouring air ambulance teams and students from paramedic, medical and nursing backgrounds. There is also collaboration with inter-agency colleagues, including HM Coastguard search and rescue, the fire and rescue service, police firearms and hazardous area response teams (HART). Intense and challenging simulated training exercises are developed, which demonstrate the different working methods and the various types of equipment carried by the different parties. All of these engagements increase understanding and awareness of the air ambulance crew's capabilities, which goes a long way towards improving a patient's experience.

Interaction with hospitals is also essential. Collaboration between the emergency department and intensive care unit of receiving hospitals means that air ambulance and hospital staff can open lines of communication, which allows for a better understanding of each other's expectations when a critically ill or injured patient arrives at hospital, whether by road or by air. This can also play a significant role when a patient needs to be transferred from one hospital to another.

Third parties who are directly involved in

BELOW **Winch training with Coastguard Rescue AW169 based at Portland in Dorset.**

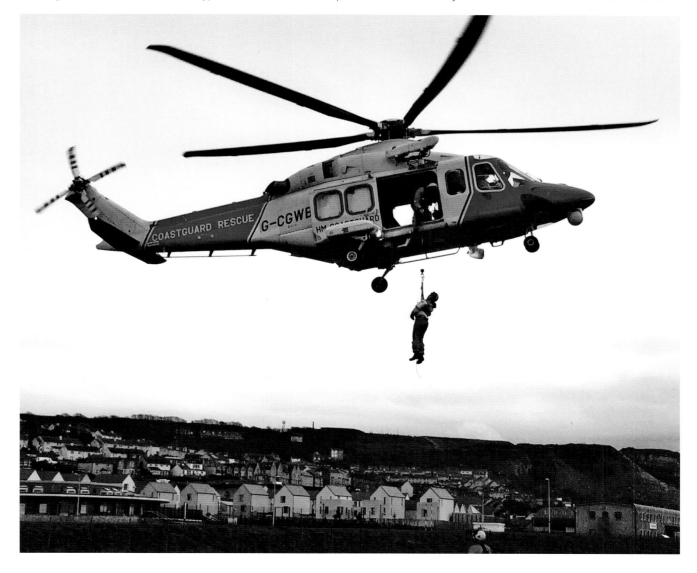

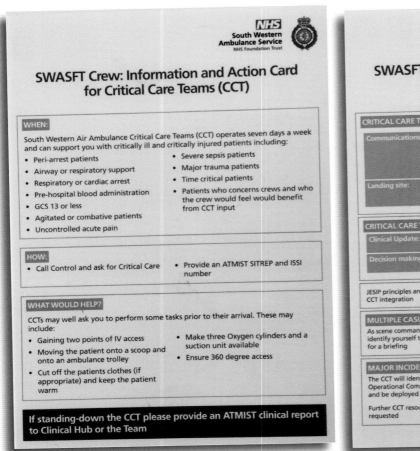

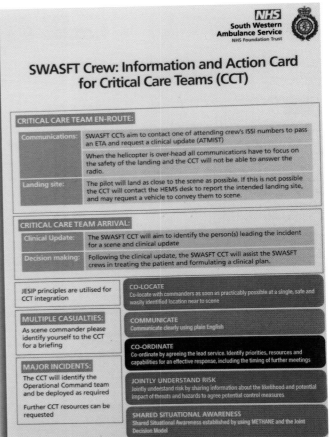

ABOVE DSAA uses prompt cards, which explain to outside colleagues what the critical care team can help with, what could be done to facilitate the patient's onward treatment pathways, and how the patient can be packaged.

patient rescue or care are invited to attend monthly clinical governance meetings to discuss cases and share knowledge to improve patient care. Everyone who has been involved in an incident directly can come to discuss the case in order to learn from it. 'It's a reflective process to see how patient care can be improved,' explains Neil. When the different crews come together, they can explain their part of the incident prior to the air ambulance's arrival – DSAA's clinicians don't always get to hear about this part as they are often absent from the debrief because they are transporting the patient away.

Closing the feedback loop on cases is an integral part of the programme. 'Crews should feel that when DSAA attended their incident, we listened to what they had to say, listened

to their plan, involved them in every aspect of the decision-making and then gave feedback on how the patient did, closing the circle,' says Neil. This means including everyone who was directly or remotely involved – such as the 999 call handler – if it's possible to do so.

After an incident, members of the DSAA crew will send personalised emails to the emergency crew that attended the incident, thanking them for their hard work, letting them know the positive gains that their interventions made and giving them feedback, if they can, about how the patient fared in hospital. For Neil, the most important part of that email is asking them to contact DSAA if they have any questions, suggestions or feedback. This more informal route to obtaining feedback provides an opportunity for two individuals to discuss how things went, rather than become bogged down with an organisation-level communication.

The DSAA crew is often attending perhaps the worst incident or illness that a paramedic will ever see in their career. 'None of us know how we will react until we are there,' says Neil. 'We are part of the supportive network and can help with the post-trauma counselling process by clarifying any points that might be causing angst.'

The overarching goal is that the patient is well looked after and safe. DSAA firmly believes that outreach has been instrumental in building trust, increasing knowledge and saving lives. During the 2013–2018 period, DSAA saw a 60% increase in the number of patients it treated, with no changes to the process of clinical tasking. Prior to the outreach programme, the number of patients treated by DSAA was static, yet because of the patient advocacy that the programme provided, hundreds of additional patients benefited from care delivered by DSAA.

CRITICAL CARE PRACTITIONER: NEIL BIZZELL

Neil's interest in emergency medicine was first sparked by his father joining the ambulance service as an ambulance technician and his neighbour becoming one of the first paramedics on the London Air Ambulance. Neil joined the London Ambulance Service in 1999 as an ambulance technician and was based at Waterloo Ambulance Station for two years, before qualifying as a paramedic in 2002 and moving to Westminster Ambulance Station, where he stayed for a decade. During this time he was seconded onto the rapid response vehicle (RRV) that operates around London's West End.

Neil's ambition had always been to work on the London HEMS, based at the Royal London Hospital in Whitechapel and, in 2006, he underwent a tough selection process and managed to secure a nine-month secondment onto London's Air Ambulance. His work there was very varied, as the rota may include a few days on the helicopter, a day in the RRV and a day or two in the control room. London's Air Ambulance uses clinical dispatch, so part of the paramedic's role is to spend some time in the control room identifying appropriate calls for the crew to attend.

Once the secondment finished, Neil returned to Westminster before moving down to Dorset with his family in 2011 and joining SWASFT in Bournemouth. In 2015 the opportunity arose to join DSAA's Critical Care Practitioner Programme and shortly afterwards, the secondment at DSAA became available.

'With such a broad range of rural and urban communities, plus the different landscapes, a helicopter really comes into its own,' says Neil. 'We don't just attend critically injured patients but critically ill ones as well, so we care for people with asthma, anaphylaxis, sepsis, respiratory illness and a host of other conditions.'

Neil was responsible for setting up DSAA's outreach programme, part of which involves joint training with the police, fire and rescue services and HM Coastguard to understand each other's capabilities as well as their limitations. 'This is really important,' says Neil. 'In most industries you have an expectation of what your colleagues can do. For us, the time to find out each other's capabilities and limitations is not when we are attending the scene of an incident.'

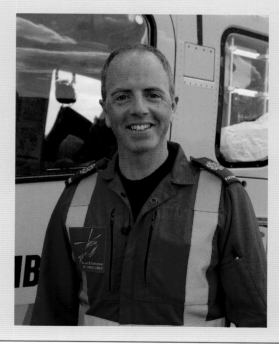

LEFT Neil Bizzell, DSAA Critical Care Practitioner and head of the outreach programme.

The counties of Dorset and Somerset have a broad range of rural and urban communities, as well as different landscapes and more than 120 miles (193km) of coastline. DSAA doesn't just attend critically injured patients but those who are critically ill as well, who may be suffering from a range of conditions, including asthma, anaphylaxis, sepsis, cardiac problems and respiratory illness. While an air ambulance helicopter comes in useful when there are access problems, there are a number of other rescue services that are experienced in rescuing patients from precarious positions.

Hazardous Area Response Teams (HART)

South Western Ambulance Service NHS Foundation Trust has two hazardous area response teams (HART), based in Bristol and Exeter. HART paramedics have been taught specific technical rescue methods, such as working in confined spaces, at height, or during civil disturbances. They can respond to situations that arise in environments involving hazardous materials, using a range of personal protective equipment including breathing apparatus and gas-tight suits. They can be delivered to patients where safe working at height or confined space rescue is required, for example in collapsed buildings, tunnels and caves, or rooftops and industrial settings like storage tanks. HART paramedics can also deliver care to patients in situations involving flooding or people injured around rivers or lakes, as well as attending scenes where ballistic protection is required from either firearms or explosives. Usually working alongside the police and fire and rescue services, HART paramedics triage and treat casualties and also look after other emergency personnel who may have been injured during the incident.

Fire and rescue services

The UK's fire and rescue services do far more than simply putting out fires. As well as attending road traffic collisions and incidents on the railways, fire and rescue services have specialist teams that can provide a range of capabilities, including rescuing people from heights, confined spaces, water and flooded areas, as well as rescuing animals, including large animals such as horses or cattle. They have a wealth of knowledge about creating safe spaces and shoring up structures, as well as enough basic medical knowledge to start off casualty care.

Police

Police forces help to keep incident scenes safe so that the clinical crews can attend to patients. While the patient is the first priority of the attending ambulance or air ambulance crew, if the crews are able to preserve evidence to assist the police with their subsequent investigations, they will.

HM Coastguard

The coastguard rescue service is made up of volunteers and is part of HM Coastguard, which is the agency responsible for initiating and co-ordinating maritime search and rescue.

Coastguard Search And Rescue (SAR) helicopters are able to winch patients to safety, (DSAA's helicopter doesn't have a winch). On occasion, DSAA crew members have been winched down by a SAR helicopter to be with patients who have fallen from cliffs, then winched back up with the patient to the clifftop, where the air ambulance was waiting.

Volunteer coastguards sometimes come out to help secure a landing site for the air ambulance, and are all trained in technical rescue, casualty care and in a variety of search and rescue capabilities.

Royal National Lifeboat Institution (RNLI)

Dorset and Somerset are blessed with miles of coastline; some sandy, some rugged and some Jurassic, with a number of beaches that become heavily used in the summer time. With its fleet of 349 lifeboats, the RNLI is able to cover some 19,000 miles (30,500km) of UK coastline. It operates separately from the coastguard, independent of the government and, like the air ambulance services, relies on volunteers and supporters to continue operating.

There are two categories of RNLI lifeboats: all-weather lifeboats and inshore lifeboats. All-weather lifeboats can reach high speeds and be operated safely, whatever the weather. They are inherently self-righting if they capsize and are fitted with navigation, location and communication equipment. Inshore lifeboats are designed to operate closer to shore, and are used for rescues in shallower water, near cliffs or rocks and even in caves. The service also has inshore rescue hovercraft for areas such as mud flats or river estuaries, which are inaccessible to conventional RNLI lifeboats. The type of lifeboat a station has depends on geographical features, the nature of the rescues the station is usually involved in and the cover provided by neighbouring lifeboat stations.

Major incidents can sometimes involve two or three air ambulances, the police, fire and rescue crews and even the coastguard in attendance at once. Each party needs to know where the others are, so the pilots all use a specific radio channel for communicating. Knowing each other's strengths and limitations and how to combine these to work together as one team is vital. A patient's outcome can be vastly improved if the team around them is all striving in the same direction.

Bridging the gap: patient and family liaison nurses

Caring for patients involves more than just medical treatment. For many patients, once they leave the care of the air ambulance team and enter a hospital or major trauma centre, their journey is just beginning. Many of them are so badly injured or critically ill that they do not recall the events during or after the incident. Others will face a long recovery process and undergo extremely difficult mental or physical challenges as a result of their injuries or illness. They may at times feel they have insufficient information about their care or any access to support once they are discharged. Sadly, the air ambulance also attends incidents in which patients do not survive and their families will often have important questions about the care that was provided to their loved one in the pre-hospital environment.

As part of their constant efforts to deliver clinical excellence, DSAA set about looking at ways to extend its service to solve some of these problems. One of its critical care doctors, James Keegan, had previously served on London's Air Ambulance and had experienced first-hand the benefit to patients of having an additional layer of support to bridge the gap between their pre-hospital care and recovery.

In 2014, London's Air Ambulance had appointed the UK's first patient liaison nurse, Frank Chege, to help patients with their transition back to independent living. DSAA had watched this appointment and the development of the role with great interest and, in 2018, asked Frank to spend some time with its team to advise on how best to set up such a service in Dorset and Somerset.

The various hospitals that DSAA's patients are transported to cover a wide area: in the south they include University Hospital Southampton, Southampton Children's Hospital, Poole General Hospital, Bournemouth Hospital, Dorset County Hospital and Salisbury Hospital; while in the north they include Yeovil Hospital, Musgrove Park Hospital, Royal Bath Hospital, Southmead Hospital, Bristol Royal Infirmary and Bristol Children's Hospital. With patients spread widely across the two counties and limited road networks in place, DSAA decided in 2019 to create two part-time patient and family liaison nurse roles, with one to focus on the north and one on the south. Their appointments were the first of their kind in the South West region.

The role of DSAA patient and family liaison nurses Jo Petheram and Kirsty Caswell is to build and enhance relationships with the

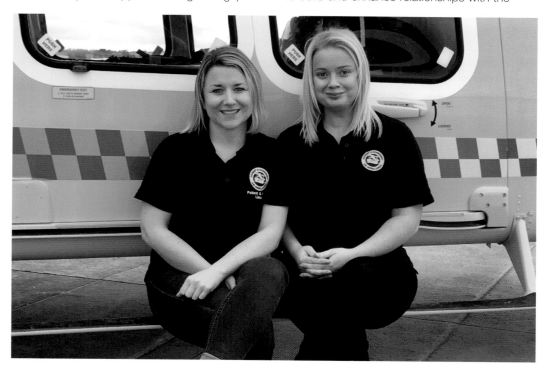

LEFT Kirsty Caswell and Jo Petheram, DSAA patient and family liaison nurses.

respective hospitals, provide support to patients who have been treated by its critical care team to help make sense of their experiences, answer patients' questions about their pre-hospital care, provide links with patient support services and other charities that are aligned with the patient's conditions, and encourage peer-support links with other similarly injured patients.

Jo and Kirsty have different but complementary backgrounds, so they brought different skillsets and knowledge to their roles. Jo is an experienced paediatric intensive care unit nurse and a member of the Regional Paediatric Retrieval Team, so she has extensive knowledge of the implications of transporting and caring for critically ill children.

Kirsty's nursing experience was gained within the emergency and critical care sector. She has several years of intensive care experience, as well as experience of working in a busy emergency department and as a resuscitation officer.

Setting up the role over such a large region has taken time. 'There are a lot of hospitals to cover, so finding the right contacts and getting the word out there has been a challenge,' says Kirsty. During their first few months, Kirsty and Jo met a number of patients to hear about their experiences. 'This has assisted us so much in identifying what needs these patients have and where the gaps in their recovery journey lie,' says Kirsty. 'One patient's family recently told us they were "haunted by the lack of knowledge" surrounding their son's incident because they had been moved away from the scene for practical reasons. We believe we have begun to fill these gaps, helping patients understand how and why they were treated and giving them the chance to talk through their incident with our clinical team.'

Part of the role is to be able to explain to patients and their families the pathway of their pre-hospital care, for example, what interventions were made at the scene, why they were treated this way, why anaesthetics were used, why they can't remember what happened or have altered memories because of the drugs they were given, and why they may have been taken to a hospital that was far from home. Jo and Kirsty can explain, debrief and reflect on their pre-hospital journey, then offer support

to patients or their relatives during their stay in hospital. Once they are discharged, they would hope to keep in touch to offer support, such as helping patients gain access to physical rehabilitation or trauma-specific counselling, as they recover.

The nurses are also working on offering a peer-support service, connecting patients who have already been through similar traumatic events with a current patient who is struggling, so they can offer hope, support and advice. 'While we do our best to understand, someone who has been through it before you is always going to be able to empathise on a deeper level,' explains Kirsty. Many links have already been forged with relevant charities, such as the Limbless Association and Headway, who can also offer emotional and practical support for patients.

While some hospitals have an intensive care follow-up service, where patients who have spent an extended time in ICU can come back and see a nurse for a follow-up clinic, this type of patient liaison role doesn't really exist elsewhere within the NHS. Jo and Kirsty are working hard to link the pre-hospital experience, to the hospital experience, to rehabilitation, through to recovery back to health.

One of the most rewarding aspects of the role, for all concerned, is when patients come back to the base to meet the crew and talk to them face to face about the incident and what has happened to them since. 'That helps us to learn from every patient that visits,' says Kirsty. 'For patients it's often therapeutic to meet the crew, as well as emotional. It helps them all to find closure.' It is also very rewarding for Jo and Kirsty to give positive feedback to the crew, who would be unable to find out about a patient's progress otherwise. For the pilots particularly, this has been a very useful development.

'From an aviation perspective you always close the loop,' says Mario Caretta, Unit Chief Pilot. 'You can see whether you have performed correctly, whether you could have done something better.' However, because of patient confidentiality rules, pilots (who are not employed by the NHS or SWASFT) have no contact with patients after they leave the scene and have previously been unable to access further information unless the patient themselves used their own initiative to get in touch. 'The patient and family liaison nurses help us to complete that loop, which helps us to improve the service,' says Mario. 'While we may not become connected to patients during an incident, you do want to know whether they survived or not.'

The liaison team will be able to achieve formal assessment of the functional outcomes of patients and feed this back into the medical system, with the aim of further closing the loop and directing improvements in care.

Sometimes, the most important service Jo and Kirsty can offer is simply to listen and provide a shoulder to cry on. 'For some of

WEATHER STATION

As you might expect, adverse weather conditions can have a significant impact on the incidents that DSAA are tasked to attend, both from the point of view of actually reaching the patient and of ensuring a safe flight. Weather information is usually obtained from local airfields, but these start to close from about 22.00h so the amount of weather information available starts to decline. When the air ambulance began flying at night, Civil Aviation Authority rules meant it was necessary for DSAA to install a weather station at its Henstridge airbase.

Produced by a company called Skyview, the weather station provides readings on visibility and cloud base data, as well as air temperature and surface wind information.

All this data can be accessed by the crew out in the field via a web page that shows data from other weather stations located across the region. This is extremely important as the weather can change rapidly from place to place on any given day.

There is little weather information available to the south of the region and the Dorchester/Portland area seems to have a unique weather pattern of its own. Because of this, DSAA's trustees agreed to purchase two more weather stations; one located at Dorset County Hospital (in Dorchester) and the other at Musgrove Park Hospital (in Taunton). These provide the crew with early warnings when bad weather is approaching and enable them to make important operational decisions.

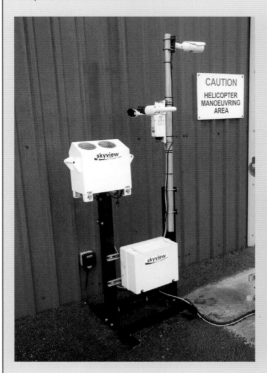

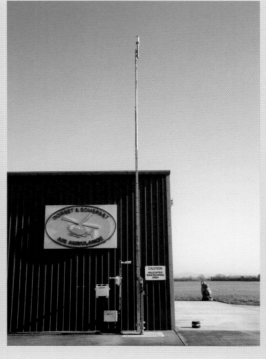

LEFT When the air ambulance began flying at night, Civil Aviation Authority rules meant it was necessary to install a weather station at DSAA's Henstridge Airfield. *(Simon Pryor)*

the patients we have met, just knowing they can talk to us is so reassuring, because their recoveries may be long and tough and at times very lonely,' says Kirsty. 'A poly-trauma patient told me recently that talking to me had changed her perspective on recovery from negative to positive, as just knowing that I would support her in achieving her goals gave her more strength to tackle them.'

Over the coming years, DSAA's patient and family liaison nurses will prove to be an important part of strengthening and enhancing the recovery of patients by supporting them as much as they can for as long as they need.

Clinical data

As with many other industries and sectors, in medicine, high-quality data is essential for improving efficiency and success rates. In order to systematically improve patient care it is necessary to feedback on care that has been provided and on the patient's outcome. 'If you never know the outcome you can't improve your patient care,' explains Phil Hyde. 'If you don't know what you did, when you did it and why, in big numbers, how can any system be improved?'

DSAA is now in the third year of development of a clinical database of pre-hospital emergency medicine (PHEM) called PHEMnet, which meets the air ambulance's specific needs. Dr Mike Eddie led the development and delivery of this innovative database. The output from PHEMnet now supports all service developments within DSAA.

The DSAA data team recognised that PHEMnet could provide a solution to the pre-hospital data collection challenges that are faced outside of Dorset and Somerset. So in creating the database, it was decided to make it scalable, in order to enable PHEMnet to support potential future national collaborative pre-hospital data collection.

PHEMnet has so far been adopted by a number of other air ambulance charities and, nationally, by the Faculty of Pre-Hospital Care of the Royal College of Surgeons of Edinburgh (RCSEd) for use by its members and as the official means of recording and assessing all PHEM trainee doctors.

'The provision of feedback within pre-hospital care has been limited by the absence of a national unifying data collection system' says Phil. 'PHEMnet provides a potential platform to enable national collation of data, analysis and feedback to inform contemporary clinical practice.'

Upgrading the aircraft

As we have seen, since the Dorset and Somerset Air Ambulance started flying almost two decades ago, the changes and

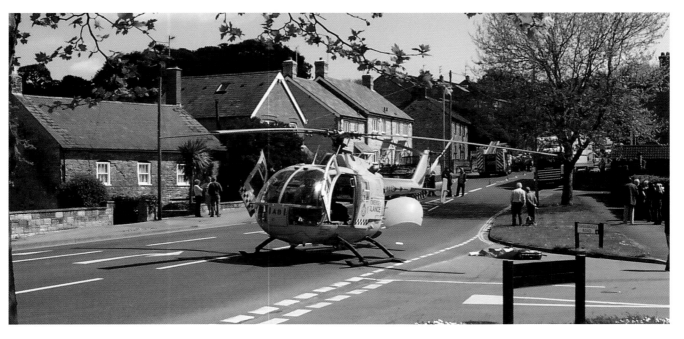

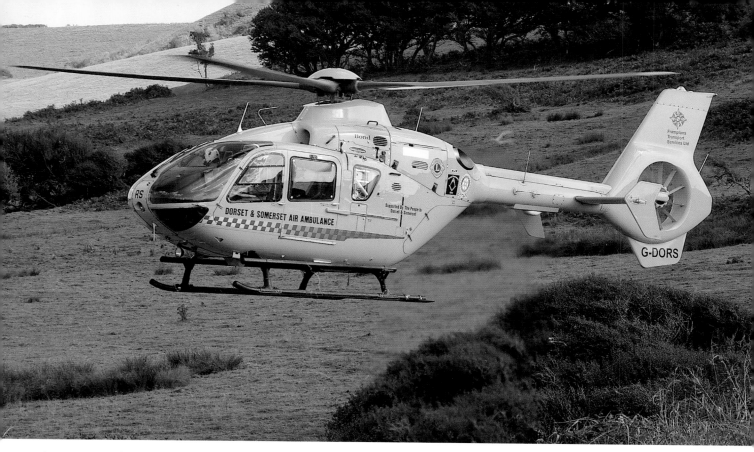

improvements in clinical care have been significant. To keep pace with these clinical developments, it has also been essential to update the aircraft to ensure the best possible air ambulance service continues to be provided.

The BO 105 served DSAA well for seven years, but in 2007 the charity decided to upgrade to a more modern aircraft, the EC135. This twin-engined utility helicopter was primarily used by the police and emergency medical services and it offered major improvements in terms of increased space, more payload and enhanced safety.

However, ten years on, developments in the clinical landscape meant that another change of aircraft was necessary. The decision was driven in part by the establishment of the NHS's National Trauma Network, which pooled expertise and facilities into major trauma centres (MTCs) around the country. These MTCs became the preferred destination for all patients suffering major trauma, but one did not exist in Dorset or Somerset, meaning that patients who would have previously been taken to the county hospitals must now be flown to Southampton, Bristol or Plymouth.

While the increased flight time to the MTCs were only a matter of minutes, those minutes

could often mean the difference between life and death for a critically ill or injured patient. This meant that DSAA paramedics needed more access to a patient en route to hospital should clinical intervention be required.

Patient benefit has always been the charity's top priority and this was the single biggest criterion in selecting the new aircraft. As this line of thought developed, the reasoning became clear: if a patient is at the centre of our thinking and in the centre of treatment on scene, then should the patient not also be at the centre of the cabin of the air ambulance?

Once this logic was applied, the choice of a successor aircraft was quite straightforward, as not all options offered the necessary cabin format to meet this requirement. Once other factors such as cost, safety and potential for night operations were also considered, it turned out that only one aircraft provided the solution to all of these needs: the AgustaWestland 169 (AW169).

It was decided that the new aircraft would not be purchased by the charity, but that it would instead invest in the AW169. This was considered to be the most cost-effective way to procure such an expensive asset – had the charity owned the aircraft, it would have had to meet the full cost of any modifications

ABOVE In 2007, DSAA upgraded to the EC135, a twin-engined utility helicopter that offered major improvements in terms of increased space, more payload and enhanced safety.
(John Edwards)

that might be required in order to preserve its eventual resale value. With aircraft parts often costing in excess of £250,000, this was a risk that the trustees felt was not justified. Under the financial arrangement, DSAA is only responsible for part of these costs.

DSAA's AW169 helicopter entered operational service on 12 June 2017; the first AW169 to enter air ambulance operational service in the UK. The culmination of years of planning and development, it was selected after an extensive evaluation process. The aircraft offered a number of outstanding characteristics and superior capabilities, include night flying, which meant it would provide an enhanced life-saving service for the people of Dorset and Somerset. As the AW169 uses the latest advances in technology, it would also be safer and easier to maintain and operate.

While the medical equipment in the AW169 is not that different to that which was carried on the EC135, the biggest difference is the increased space inside the cabin. This allows the critical care team to have complete access to a patient, which obviously provides

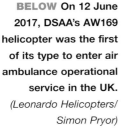

a significant benefit if a patient needs further intervention or treatment en route to hospital.

Specialist Aviation Services operates the AW169 helicopter on DSAA's behalf and the company worked closely with the clinical team to develop a medical interior that enables them to fully meet the needs of their patients. This approach meant that the AW169 had to undergo very intense scrutiny by the European Aviation Safety Agency before it could become operational.

Existing DSAA pilots underwent conversion training to the new aircraft, which included training for night Helicopter Emergency Medical Service (HEMS) missions. While they were being trained, two new pilots who had already completed their training and were qualified to undertake night missions joined the team.

At the launch, CEO Bill Sivewright said: 'It has always been the charity's aim and clear vision to pursue clinical excellence; pairing critical care teams with the outstanding capabilities of the AW169 is a natural development of that vision.'

Within a few hours of being operational, the critical care team was tasked to its first

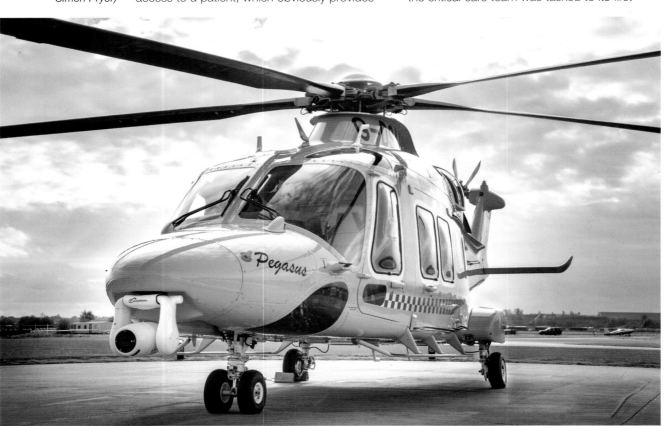

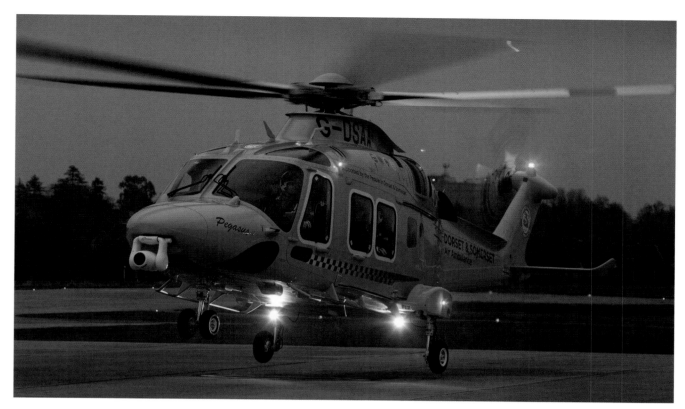

incident flying the AW169. A man who had suffered a cardiac arrest was airlifted from Dorchester to the secondary landing site near Royal Bournemouth Hospital.

In autumn 2017, DSAA launched a competition to find a name for the new aircraft. A judging panel decided on the winning entry, *Pegasus*, which was announced at the formal unveiling ceremony at the start of 2018.

Night HEMS

The AW169's night flying capabilities have enabled DSAA to provide full night HEMS missions. The team can fly directly to the patient without the need for any fixed or pre-established lighting, which is a significant advantage. Embarking on night HEMS missions meant that DSAA was able to increase the operating hours for the aircraft to 19 hours a day, to cover the period from 07.00h through to 02.00h.

Although the latest night vision technology is provided to assist the crew, flying at night does increase the overall risk levels that they face. When trying to land, new hazards are present, such as power lines or masts, which are difficult to see in the darkness.

To reduce the risk when flying at night, the crew spends time looking at computer images of possible landing sites nearby. Because the images could be out of date, or variables such as livestock may be present when the helicopter arrives on scene, two possible locations, a primary and a secondary, are chosen and closely examined for possible hazards. Only when the crew are happy and have planned their approach into the selected sites does *Pegasus* launch.

It may be unavoidable, but precious minutes are lost carrying out these vital surveys of possible night landing sites. DSAA therefore decided to create a grid of pre-surveyed landing sites across the two counties, which would enable launch with the minimum of planning and so bring its life-saving service to where it is needed with minimum delay.

The call went out to communities and individuals across Dorset and Somerset to offer DSAA the use of their field, sports pitch or playing field as potential night landing sites for the air ambulance. The criteria were: a level area of grass, tarmac or concrete measuring a minimum of 30 metres by 60 metres [100 by 200ft] (a football pitch measures 45 metres by

ABOVE Night HEMS missions meant that DSAA was able to increase its operating hours to 19 hours a day.

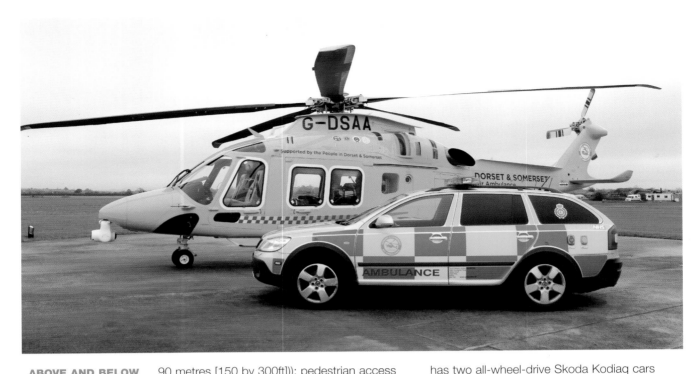

90 metres [150 by 300ft])); pedestrian access to the site; and vehicle access close by. The response was overwhelming and teams went out to survey potential sites. A number of sites were chosen and all sites will be re-evaluated annually to ensure that any changes that might affect night operations are recorded.

Rapid response vehicles

Pegasus is not always able to fly to an incident, so being able to mobilise the clinical team by road is essential. DSAA currently

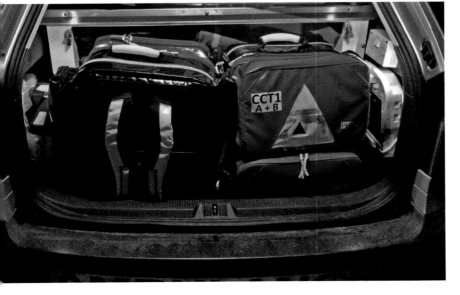

has two all-wheel-drive Skoda Kodiaq cars available to use. The whole team is trained to drive on blue lights and each team member also receives additional driving training every year. The road systems in Dorset and Somerset mean the RRVs can face long journey times and the crew could find themselves driving on blue lights for 30 minutes or more, which is challenging.

'It provides us with resilience and means we can have a car out in the field, in the biggest conurbations, acting as our eyes and ears,' says DSAA Medical Lead Phil Hyde.

Outreach is a key function of the RRVs. While having cars out on the road helps to spread the message to the public that DSAA exists, it also strengthens ties with colleagues on the ground. 'With an aircraft, you often come in, see the patient and fly away,' explains Phil. 'It can be dissociated from our ambulance service colleagues. Down on the ground, there is a lot more opportunity for communication.'

In addition to this, there are types of advanced pain relief that the ambulance service are not able to provide, or clinical decisions that might need to be made, which require a doctor. In certain situations it is not possible for a helicopter to attend, but the ambulance service is then able to request a DSAA car in order to bring a critical care team to the patient.

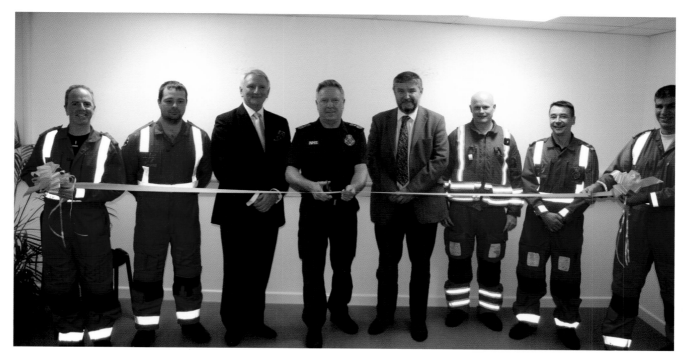

Clinical training facility

The AW169 is approximately a third larger than the EC135 it replaced, and having a bigger aircraft meant that the Dorset and Somerset Air Ambulance had to think carefully about all aspects of its operation. This included the suitability of the hangar and helipad at its Henstridge airbase, the helipads at the various hospitals in the region and, crucially, the aircraft's ability to land at incident sites.

The increased size of the aircraft did not mean that significant adjustments were required at any of the fixed sites across the two counties. However, some did need to make adjustments to cater for DSAA's new ability to conduct night operations. Night operations demand a larger helipad than daylight operations, as well as some adjustments to lighting – Royal Bournemouth Hospital was one of those to make changes to its existing helipad.

In order to fully exploit the planned development of clinical and aviation capabilities, DSAA identified the need for a modern clinical training facility and a day/night aviation planning facility, as well as the need to provide technical storage space and improved crew rest facilities. In 2015, two years before DSAA's AW169 entered service, the Chancellor of the Exchequer awarded £5 million from the fund established from LIBOR fines to support air ambulance

charities across the UK, which was distributed by the Association of Air Ambulances Charity. A gift of £250,000 enabled DSAA to upgrade its operational facilities to meet any planned and possible future developments.

'We didn't have a formal briefing facility for aviation and, as the service moved into night operations, that would become an absolute requirement,' explains CEO Bill Sivewright. The 50-seat clinical training facility has also been a huge step forward, as it enables the whole team to come in for in-house training, governance meetings and case reviews, as well as being used for outreach training for student paramedics, doctors and nurses and other visitors.

All work had to be completed so that the hangar was ready to receive the new AW169 helicopter, and coincided with the recruitment of the new paramedics and doctors that enabled DSAA to extend its operating hours from 12 to 19 hours per day. Once the charity secured funding for the project, the work began on remodelling and took approximately eight weeks to complete. The project was managed by Babcock International.

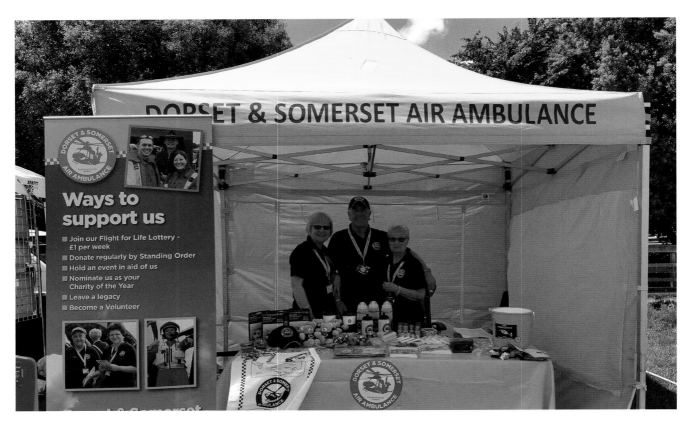

ABOVE The DSAA's merchandising stall, manned by a team of volunteers, can be found at many local events in the Dorset/ Somerset area.

Funding and fundraising

Operating 19 hours a day, 365 days a year doesn't come cheap: the clinical and aviation costs alone are just under £4 million a year. In 2017/18, DSAA was called to 1,197 incidents, an almost two-fold increase since 2013. Despite an almost doubling of costs, the increase in incidents responded to means that the average cost of each mission has stayed relatively constant at around £3,000.

For the first few years of service, the flying costs of DSAA were met by the AA as part of the £14 million grant for air ambulances, while medical costs were met by the regional ambulance services. Like its counterparts throughout the UK, the charity receives no direct funding from the government or the National Lottery. Even though DSAA works hand-in-glove with the government-funded South Western Ambulance Service NHS Foundation Trust, it is because of that very relationship that DSAA is unable to apply for a National Lottery grant because the rules do not allow them to 'top up' government spending.

VOLUNTEERS: A HELPING HAND

Most charities rely heavily on the support of volunteers in order to function effectively. DSAA has a team of more than 100 dedicated individuals who perform a wide range of duties on the charity's behalf, covering a staggering 2,636 square miles across the two counties.

These duties include giving talks on how the charity works, providing support at events, manning information and merchandise stalls, visiting fundraisers to thank them and collect money raised, and helping to organise collection boxes.

Currently, the time put in by volunteers amounts to some 5,000 hours of support that would otherwise have to be provided by paid staff. This has significant monetary value, as well as giving the extra benefit of boosting the charity's profile within local communities. Many events simply wouldn't be possible without the generosity of each and every volunteer.

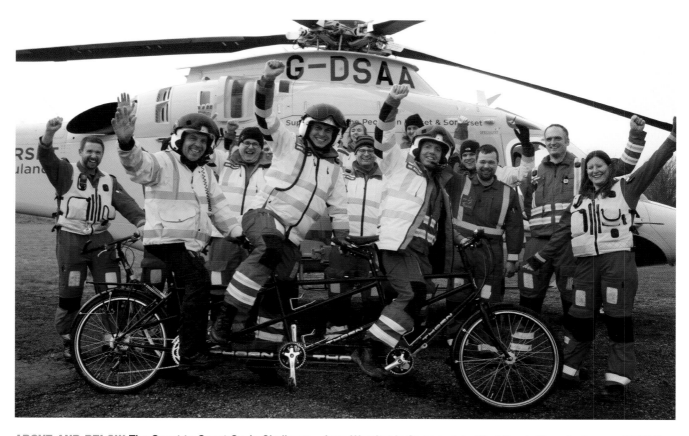

ABOVE AND BELOW The Coast to Coast Cycle Challenge – from Watchet in Somerset, to West Bay in Dorset – is one of DSAA's most popular annual fundraising events, involving some 600 cyclists. The crew has taken part for a number of years.

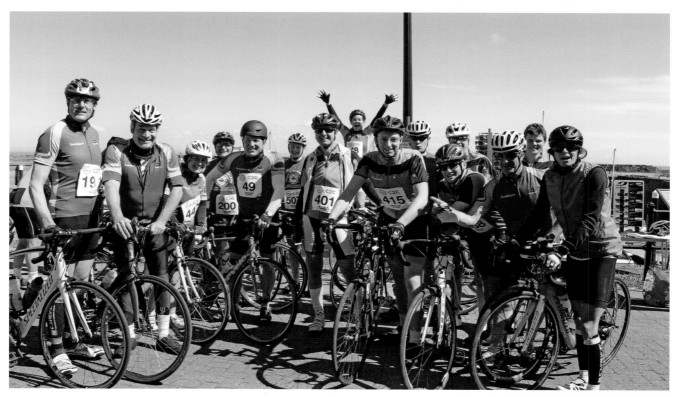

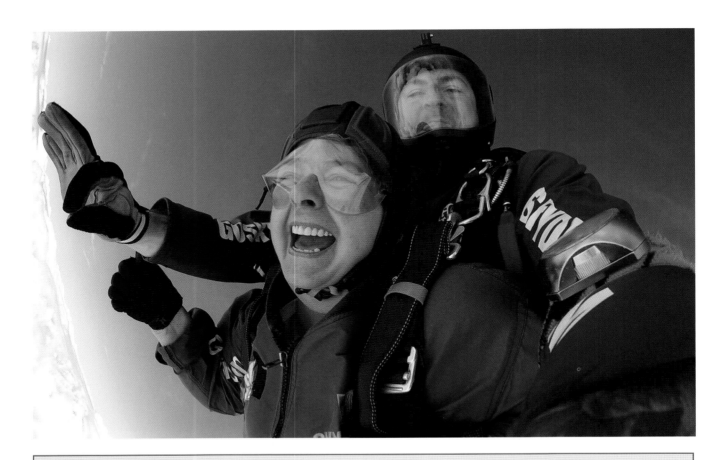

THE FLIGHT FOR LIFE LOTTERY

Running a year-round air ambulance service across two counties comes at a steep price. The Dorset and Somerset Air Ambulance needs around £4 million per year to stay operational and the Flight for Life Lottery, with its 86,000 members, is the service's main source of funding.

Held weekly, the lottery costs £1 per week to join and all money raised goes directly to the charity. Customers are under no obligation to keep playing and can join for any time period. Each Friday, a computer randomly selects the winners and a top prize of £1,000, plus a number of other cash and consolation prizes, are awarded. The prize money does not roll over – meaning money is awarded every week, with winners being notified by the charity and their prize money being paid directly into their bank accounts. As well as the weekly computerised draw, there are two grand draws in the summer and at Christmas.

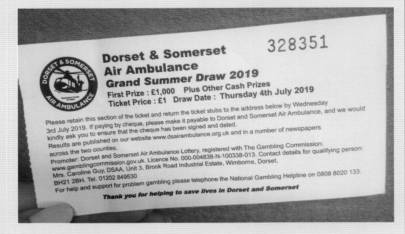

The Flight for Life Lottery was launched in 2000 and DSAA's canvassing team work hard to recruit new lottery members by visiting homes, attending events and drumming up support in supermarkets across the two counties. The lottery is licensed and regulated by the Gambling Commission and any person aged 16 or over who resides in the UK can take part.

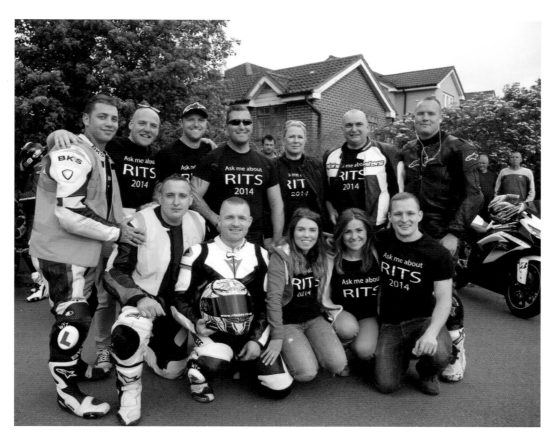

Fundraising is therefore critical to the continued operation of the air ambulance and DSAA is reliant on the generosity of the general public and private sector to provide financial support. The charity is entirely responsible for raising the necessary funds to keep the air ambulance flying and has gone to considerable effort to establish a fundraising model that is resilient, rather than be pressed into short-term gains. Its focus is on establishing and maintaining the broadest base of support, while supporting those who fundraise on its behalf.

'Some organisations operate on a more "corporate-focused" model,' explains Bill. 'They have a lower volume of givers but higher value. We are the exact opposite. We have worked on the principle of getting a broad level of support with whatever people wish to give.' This approach was tested during the last recession in 2008/09, but fundraising remained steady and enabled the charity to continue its growth. 'In times of recession and hardship it's not personal giving that falls away, it's corporate giving,'

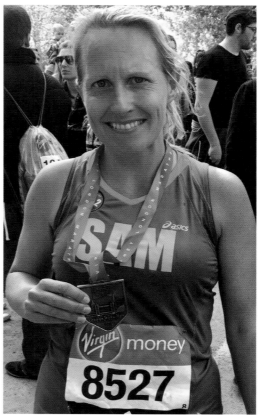

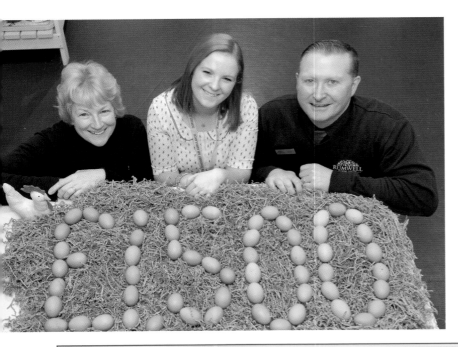

says Bill. 'People are almost inclined on a personal level to give more, it's an inverse rule really.' He describes the charity's fundraising policy as being extremely benign. 'Our advertising centres on what we do and what we deliver,' he says. 'If people want to support that, that's great.'

DSAA's Flight for Life Lottery provides far and away the largest source of funds. It is now one of the most successful society lotteries in the country and one of the most gratifying elements of this for DSAA is that many of its members simply regard it as regular giving.

While it represents a significant portion of

LEFT Rumwell Farm in Somerset has hosted a series of fundraising initiatives for DSAA.

LOTTERY MANAGER: CAROLINE GUY

Caroline joined DSAA in 2005 from Barclay's Bank, and worked alongside the charity's first lottery manager, Gareth Williams. Gareth was instrumental in growing the lottery from the very beginning and when he retired in 2017, Caroline took over his role.

With several hundred members dropping out of the lottery each week, an effective canvassing strategy is essential. A company called Lottery Fundraising Services (LFS) supplies DSAA with a canvassing team, which is pre-vetted, trained and managed. At least eight canvassers work five or more days a week. 'These canvassers work exclusively for the charity and many have worked with us for a long time, a loyalty which is fairly unusual in charity canvassing,' says Caroline. LFS has a strict induction process, part of which involves training its canvassers to be Dementia Friends, which helps them identify people in this group and to take additional care to act appropriately when faced with someone vulnerable.

DSAA must demonstrate to the Fundraising Regulator that it polices the actions of its canvassers. 'We are constantly monitoring the team in order to maintain the highest standard of fundraising behaviour,' says Caroline. She attends regular six-monthly training sessions and makes welcome calls to new members to make sure that canvassers were friendly and polite, presented their ID, wore branded clothing and didn't apply any undue pressure.

Canvassers either go door-to-door or work from supermarkets across the two counties. The easiest and most cost-effective way of joining the lottery is by direct debit, so canvassers use an LFS Datasafe machine,

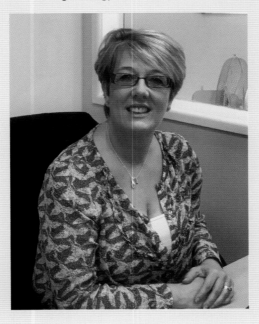

RIGHT Lottery Manager Caroline Guy.

the charity's annual income, the Flight for Life Lottery is only one of the fundraising activities that it undertakes. The charity campaigns tirelessly for local groups, businesses and individuals to participate in a range of activities. From holding relatively small-scale events such as coffee mornings or jumble sales, to taking part in recycling initiatives, helping with collection boxes or even organising a sponsored parachute jump, the ways in which the public can help are numerous.

Individuals or organisations who want to help can use the fundraising tool on DSAA's website, which enables its supporters to set up their own fundraising page. This is hugely

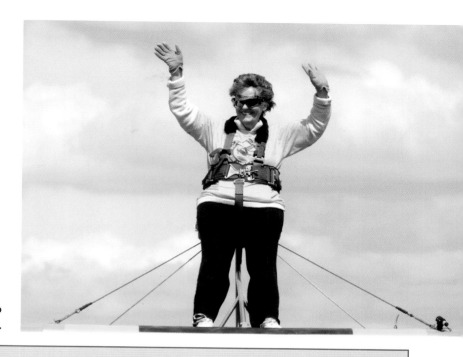

RIGHT Eileen Hall did a sponsored wing walk to celebrate her 70th birthday.

which is a secure method of taking customer details. As soon as any data is input and stored onto the device, it is encrypted to a very high level and remains encrypted during transmission and storage on the cloud server until it is imported into DSAA's database. 'If anyone was able to get hold of the machine they wouldn't be able to access any data,' explains Caroline.

'Datasafe machines are a much more effective way of gathering details,' she continues. 'In the early days, things were all done on paper, so you had paper mandates out in the field, which were not secure. You were also reliant on being able to read a canvasser's writing and whether they had written down the data correctly.' The Datasafe machines are loaded with the Royal Mail postcode file, so canvassers just tap in a postcode and select the correct address from a dropdown box. They also contain the sort code directory, which is loaded with every sort code and account number that exists, so when a customer gives their bank details the canvasser can validate and if necessary correct those details on the spot. 'This way of working is a lot safer from the customer's point of view, as well as being more carbon efficient,' says Caroline.

Society lotteries have transformed over the

years and they are the biggest sustainable income stream for many charities around the UK, large and small. Canvassers have an important role to play in this success and they probably see and speak to more members of the public than anyone else who works for DSAA. 'We find people aren't really doing it to win the prize but to support the charity,' says Caroline.

BELOW Lottery Canvasser Charlie.

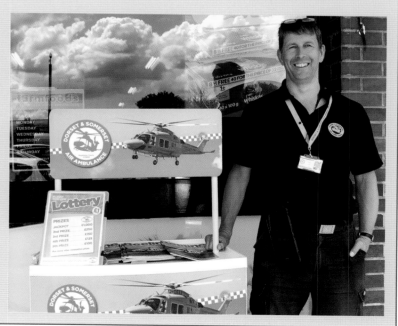

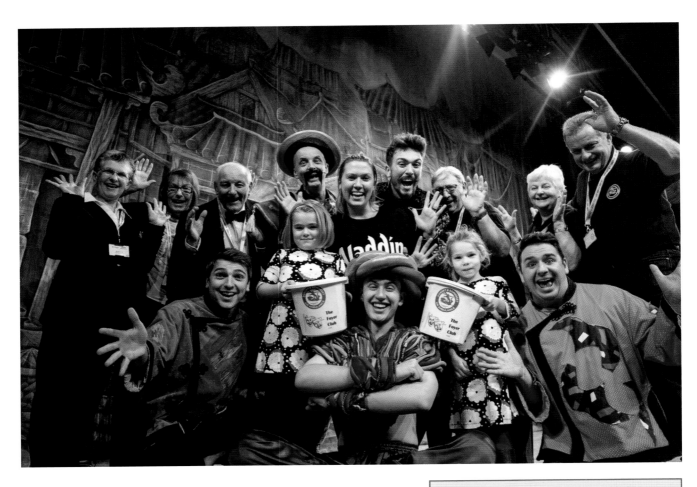

ABOVE Octagon Theatre in Yeovil raised £4,449 via bucket collections, which took place at the end of each pantomime performance of *Aladdin*.

beneficial to the charity, as it doesn't have to pay any commission fees to third-party fundraising websites.

Every penny raised makes a huge difference and enables the air ambulance to continue its life-saving work. The charity is always on hand to fully support its fundraisers, either by providing fundraising merchandise, promoting events on its website, sending along a representative or simply by providing advice and guidance.

Full training is also provided for DSAA's army of volunteers who represent the charity at events, service its collection boxes at over 2,000 outlets across the two counties, attend cheque presentations on the charity's behalf and carry out talks at a variety of clubs and groups. Hundreds of supporter-led events are held each year.

LEGACIES

In recent years, DSAA has seen an increase in the number of people who have chosen to remember the charity in their wills.

For many people, the thought of preparing a will is something they'd rather not think about and is usually put off. However, the process of making a new will or updating an existing one can actually be very straightforward. DSAA always recommends that supporters consult a solicitor to help them and it has created a booklet that outlines the process, to help supporters get started.

'For many people the content of their will is a very private matter,' says Richard Popper, DSAA Trustee. 'Advising us of your future intentions means that we can make sure we keep you up to date with our latest news and developments and it also helps us plan for the future.'

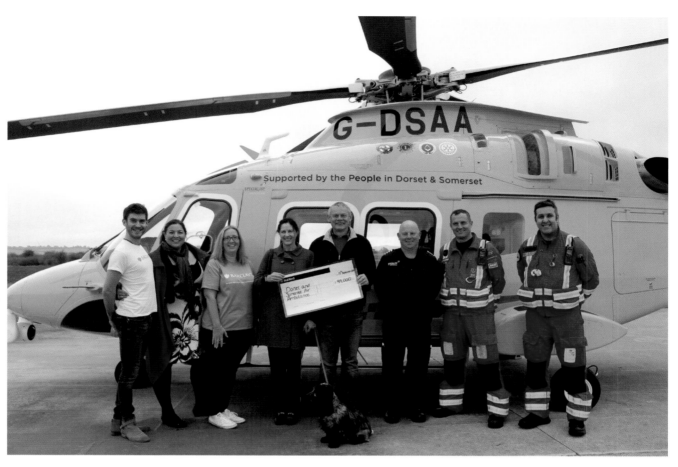

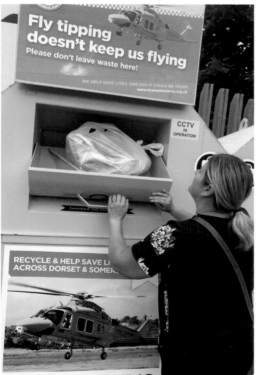

ABOVE Actor Martin Clunes and his wife Philippa organise the annual Buckham Fair, which has chosen **DSAA** as its beneficiary charity on a number of occasions.

LEFT From holding relatively small-scale events such as coffee mornings, to taking part in recycling initiatives or even organising a sponsored parachute jump, the ways in which the public raises funds are numerous.

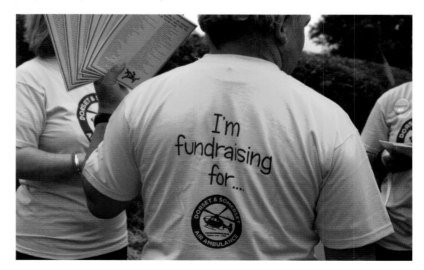

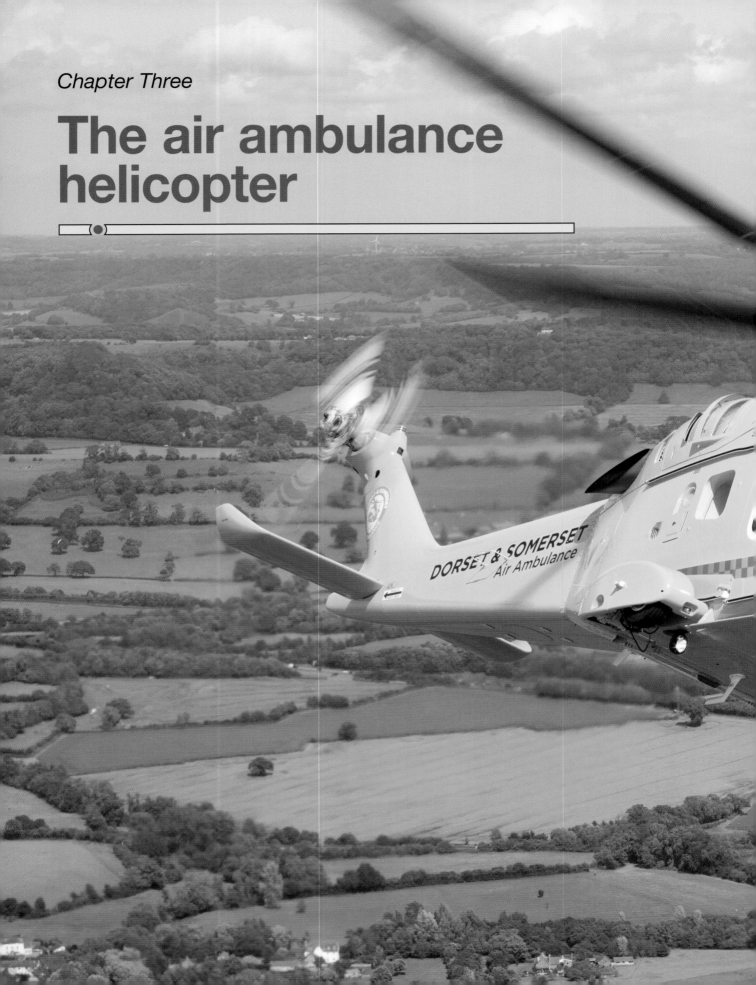

Chapter Three

The air ambulance helicopter

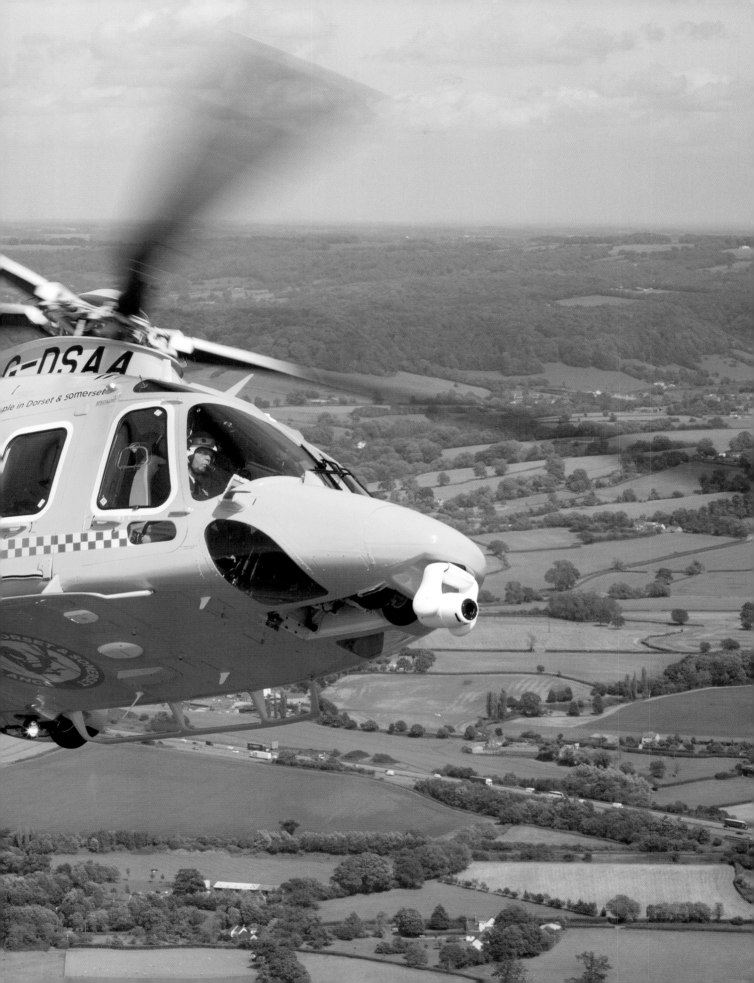

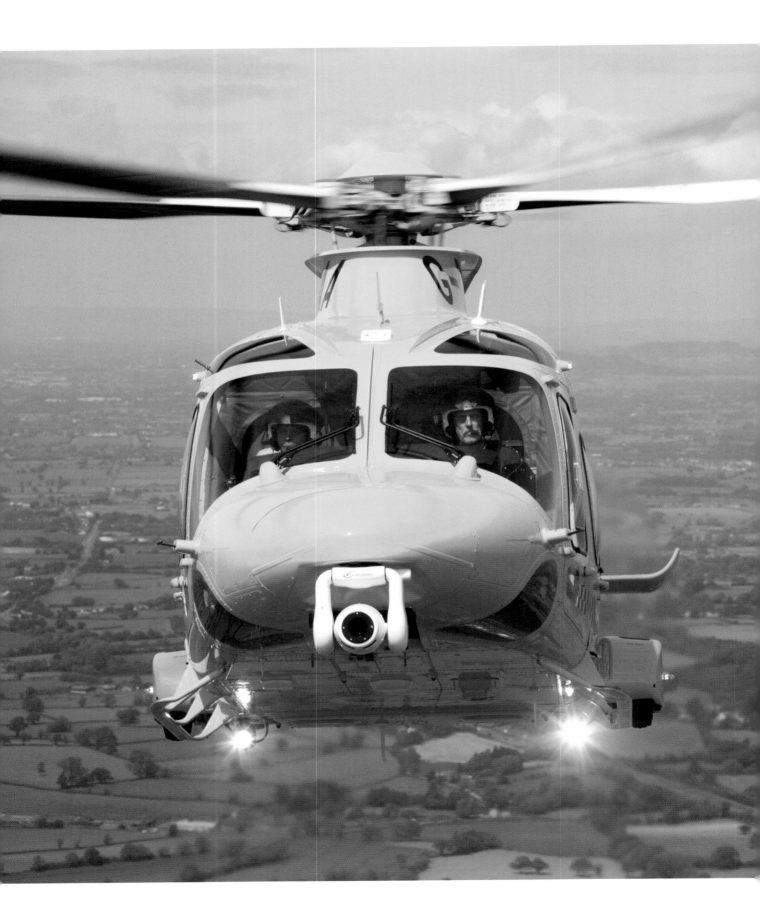

How a helicopter flies

In order for any aircraft to fly, it needs to generate lift in order to overcome the force of gravity and get off the ground. Lift can be explained by something called the Bernoulli principle. In the mid-1700s, a Swiss scientist called Daniel Bernoulli discovered that an increase in the speed of any fluid (air is a fluid because it flows and can change shape) goes hand in hand with a decrease in its pressure. Fast-moving air equals low air pressure, while slow-moving air equals high air pressure. If you imagine an aeroplane's wing in flight, the fast-moving air over the top lowers the pressure, so the slower-moving, high-pressure air beneath it pushes it up.

The main rotor blades of a helicopter are effectively its wings and they rotate at extremely high speeds, generating an enormous downdraft of air, which pushes the helicopter upwards. So, while an aeroplane typically generates lift while moving forwards, using the aerodynamic nature of its wings, the high-speed spinning of a helicopter's rotors enables it to create lift without forward motion, hence its ability to take off and land vertically.

Once the aircraft gets off the ground, Newton's third law of motion comes into play: for every action, there is an equal and opposite reaction. When the main rotor blades spin, a force called torque is generated. This force would make the fuselage spin in the opposite direction to the rotation of the rotor blades, meaning the helicopter would spin out of control, were it not for the tail rotor. The tail rotor is mounted perpendicularly and generates thrust to counteract the torque of the main rotor.

Getting airborne is all well and good, but for the pilot to achieve controlled flight, they have to co-ordinate three main controls: cyclic stick, collective lever and yaw pedals. The cyclic is the central control stick that controls the main

OPPOSITE AND BELOW Helicopters can move vertically up and down, as well as being able to hover. They are also more agile in the air and can fly sideways or backwards, meaning they can take off and land without using a runway. *(Richard Preston)*

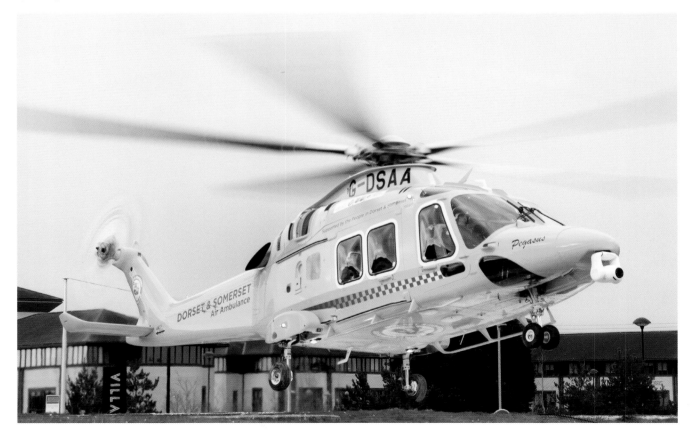

rotor, which changes the helicopter's direction of movement by altering the angle of pitch of each of the main rotor blades independently. By using a series of small movements and changes in pressure, the pilot uses the cyclic to keep the helicopter centred and can control its movement and direction. The collective, a lever that is usually located to the left of the pilot, increases the pitch on all blades simultaneously, generating and controlling lift. Unsurprisingly, the collective is raised to increase lift and lowered to decrease lift and enable the helicopter to descend.

The AW169 has a Full Authority Digital Engine Control (FADEC) system, which means once the engines have been started and the engine control levers are set to flight mode the power control is automatic, keeping the rotational speed of the rotors within the correct operating range in order to produce enough

lift to fly. Yaw control is achieved by operating the tail rotor; foot pedals operate the tail rotor blades collectively and make the helicopter yaw to the left or right.

Operating an AW169 in the air ambulance role

Helicopters are well-suited to the emergency medical services role, as their rotors allow them to function in ways other aircraft cannot. While an aeroplane needs to move forward at great speed in order to achieve lift, a helicopter can move straight up and down, as well as being able to hover. Helicopters are also more agile in the air and can fly sideways or backwards, meaning they can take off and land without using a runway, which is ideal when collecting a patient from a tricky-to-reach site or delivering them to a small hospital landing pad.

The demands on an air ambulance and its crew are intense and it is essential to have an aircraft that can meet all the day-to-day challenges of running such a service. The outstanding capabilities of the AW169 provided

BELOW The larger cabin size means the AW169 can carry additional clinical staff, which improves the range and level of care a patient will receive in transit. *(John Emery)*

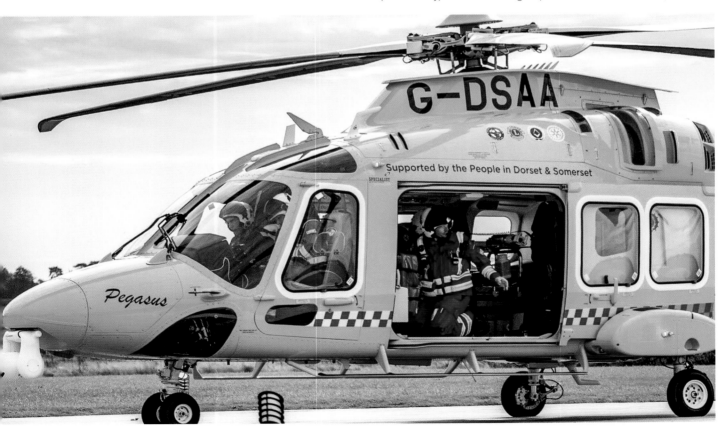

a good fit with DSAA's pursuit of clinical excellence. Patient benefit is the service's top priority and this provided the single biggest motivation in selecting the aircraft.

The AW169 is the first all-new helicopter in its weight class in more than 30 years. The 4.8 tonne aircraft is a versatile, twin-engine, light intermediate category helicopter, but with large helicopter technology. A number of new technology features are incorporated in the rotor system, engines, avionics, transmission and electric power generation and distribution systems. Currently, it is the best-selling helicopter in its class for a wide range of applications, including emergency medical services, corporate/VIP transport, offshore transport and law enforcement. As you would expect, it is fully compliant with all the latest certification standards and has inherent architectural safety features. It can also be fully customised inside in order to undertake an emergency medical services role.

Suited to both primary and secondary Helicopter Emergency Medical Services (HEMS) missions, the AW169 can accommodate one or two stretchers, either longitudinally or transversally, which is especially important for operations where in-flight stretcher recovery is required. The cabin can also accommodate wheeled stretchers and undergoes a custom medical fit, where it can be configured with a full suite of advanced clinical and life-support equipment.

For the Dorset and Somerset Air Ambulance, the AW169 helicopter offered a number of benefits that set it apart from other aircraft in the sector. 'Our ambitions and clinical aspirations determined a particular requirement from whichever aircraft we selected,' explains DSAA CEO Bill Sivewright. 'The capabilities and flexibility offered by the AW169 made it a clear winner and in our view it was the only aircraft which fully met our criteria. Another major plus in selecting a new mark of aircraft is that you are taking advantage of the latest advances

BELOW Medical procedures that may once have taken place on the ground can now take place in flight, saving valuable time. *(Leonardo Helicopters/Simon Pryor)*

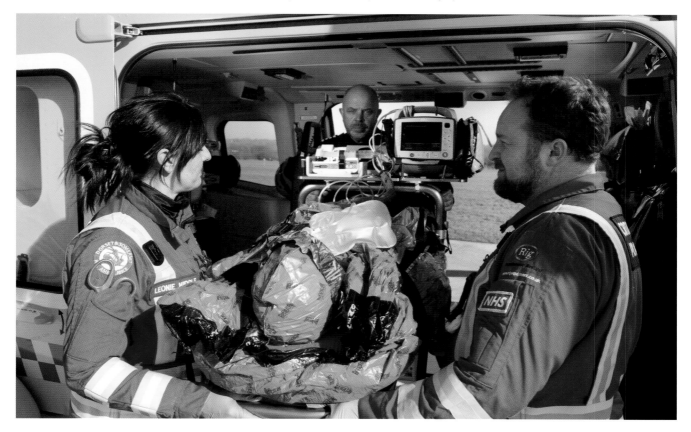

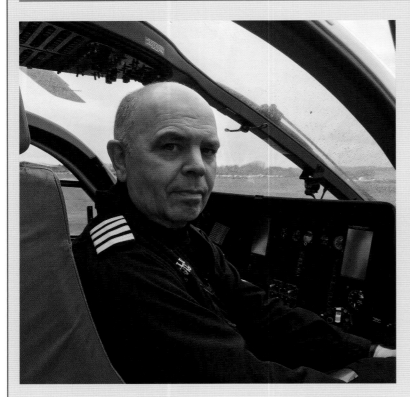

Carretta works every third day when the pilots are around, and covers their shifts when they are away on leave, so he works the same number of days but with no set pattern.

Mario joined DSAA in 2017. One of three DSAA pilots with a military background, Mario spent 27 years in the Royal Navy, based at Royal Naval Air Station Yeovilton in South West England, flying Sea King helicopters in the troop-carrying role. When he left the Royal Navy he became a test pilot, testing helicopters on ships around the world, before having to apply for a civilian pilot's licence (unlike other countries, the UK gives little recognition of military flying experience). Once he had his civilian licence, Mario joined Babcock as a floating pilot, working on various UK air ambulance bases before taking on the role at DSAA.

As an air ambulance pilot, Mario's primary responsibility is the safety of the crew, the patient and those on the ground. 'You want to help the patient but you can't cut corners and rush things,' he explains. 'If flying conditions deteriorate, or the weather is marginal, sometimes we do have to turn back. I'm all for trying, but sometimes you just know it's not possible. You need to move as quickly as you can, as safely as you can.'

Dorset and Somerset Air Ambulance has one unit chief pilot and three pilots, who are all recruited, trained and employed by Specialist Aviation Services (SAS), the operator of DSAA's AW169. The pilots are on a set roster of five days on, four days off. Unit Chief Pilot Mario in technology. That means that it is safer and easier to maintain and operate.'

The larger cabin size gives the AW169 the capability to carry additional clinical staff, thereby improving the range and level of care a patient will receive in transit. Procedures that may once have taken place on the ground can now take place in flight, saving valuable time – the more you can do for the patient while they are on board, the earlier you can leave the scene of an incident and the sooner the patient reaches hospital. And because of the increased fuel capacity and power capability, the crew can also travel from one call to another, rather than returning to base to refuel, meaning that more incidents can be covered during the course of a shift.

The two-pilot operation allows for night flying, which can significantly increase the number of patients that can be attended to on any given day. During daylight hours, DSAA operates as a single-pilot operation, but all the doctors and Critical Care Practitioners (CCPs) are also trained as crew members. At night, an extra CCP joins the team and sits in the front left-hand seat, acting as a Technical Crew Member (TCM) by assisting the pilot with cockpit duties on the way to an incident. This includes helping with navigation, reading out heights, speeds and rates of descent, as well as aiding the pilot's general awareness – everything a co-pilot would do, except actually fly. For DSAA, this method of working has proved more efficient than employing two pilots, as once the

HEMS PILOT: DAN KITTERIDGE

Dan Kitteridge joined the Royal Navy in 1997 and flew helicopters for them for 16 years. Ever since childhood, he had wanted to be a pilot and join the armed forces, so was delighted to end up serving in the Fleet Air Arm, where DSAA Unit Chief Pilot Mario Carretta was one of his instructors, teaching Dan how to fly the Sea King Mk 4. Stationed at Yeovilton, Dan flew all over the world, serving two operational tours in Iraq, as well as serving in Bosnia and flying all over Europe and the US.

This varied career gave him experience in a number of different flying environments, including the desert and the Arctic, which was good preparation for some of the challenges faced in a HEMS environment. He left the Royal Navy in 2013 and, having had a lot of night-flying experience, found himself around at the right time, as many air ambulances were starting to fly at night. He joined Kent, Surrey and Sussex Air Ambulance, flying out of Redhill, before joining DSAA in 2017.

Dan was able to draw on the experience he gained in the armed services and apply it to how he approaches different landing sites in different conditions at different times of day.

'One of the attractions of HEMS is not knowing what you will be faced with on

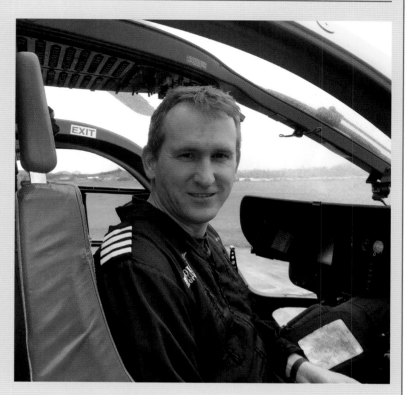

a day-to-day basis,' says Dan. 'It's a real privilege to work with this team. You wouldn't necessarily put together the two very different specialisations of aviation and medicine, but it's humbling to see what can happen when you do.'

ABOVE Dan Kitteridge, DSAA HEMS pilot.

helicopter has landed, the TCM is then also on hand to assist with clinical duties, rather than simply waiting with the aircraft.

The range and power capability of the AW169 is exceptional. With previous aircraft, the crew had to constantly think about fuel and weight, especially during the summer months when higher temperatures mean the engines produce less power, reducing the maximum take-off weight. On a really hot day with a large team, crew members sometimes had to be left at the scene in order for the helicopter to lift the patient. It was also sometimes necessary to burn off fuel before they could carry a patient and this is no longer an issue – in fact, it is now possible to take passengers, such as trainees or parents of child patients, if need be.

The fuel capacity and power capability of the AW169 allows the crew to fly from incident to incident – as many as three incidents back to back – meaning the service is now reaching twice as many patients as before. The first four AW169 air ambulances to enter service in the UK in their first year of service performed nearly 3,000 life-saving missions and flew more than 2,200 hours. Since 2015, DSAA has doubled the number of missions undertaken from 600 to 1,200, increasing its flying hours from 30–40 to 40–60 hours a month.

Pegasus, DSAA's AW169, entered into service in June 2017 and at the time of writing in 2019, 2018/19 had seen the service tasked to 1,259 incidents, treating 847 patients.

**AW169 main exterior
dimensions.**

(Leonardo Helicopters)

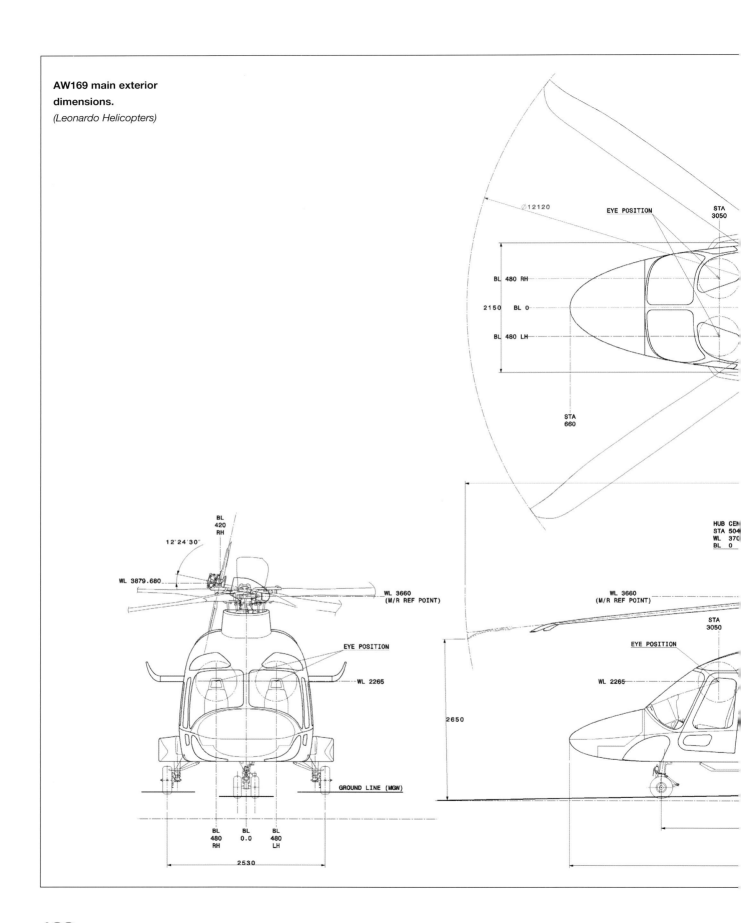

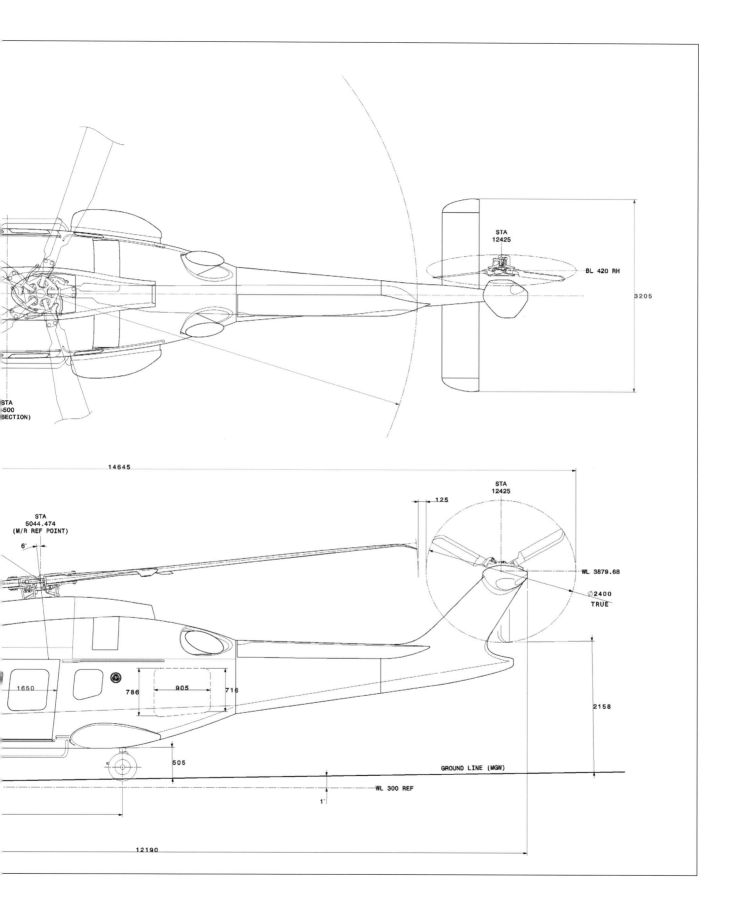

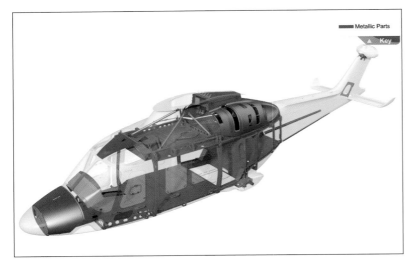

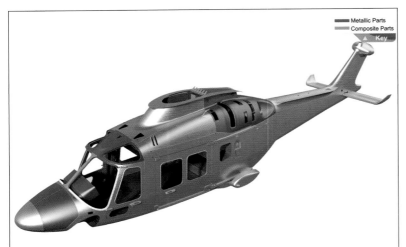

Anatomy of an AW169

Airframe
Fuselage

The AW169 airframe structure is constructed using a combination of aluminium alloy and composite materials, which makes it strong and provides resistance to fatigue and corrosion. The composite parts are primarily constructed in carbon fibre. Both the airframe and the cockpit are resistant to bird strikes and the aircraft is designed to withstand emergency landings. The airframe comprises primary structures designed to handle the loads encountered both when flying (aerodynamic loads) and on the ground (static loads and loads imposed when moving the helicopter or carrying out maintenance, for example). The AW169's fuselage is divided into four main sections: forward fuselage; centre fuselage; rear fuselage; and tail unit and tail plane.

The forward fuselage includes the radome (a weatherproof enclosure or covering that protects

TOP AND LEFT The airframe structure is manufactured using a combination of aluminium alloy and composite materials.
(Leonardo Helicopters)

BELOW Airframe primary structures.
(Leonardo Helicopters)

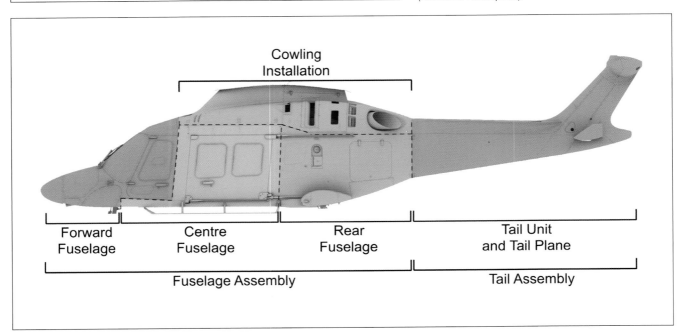

the radar antenna), the nose avionic bay (which houses the electronic systems) and the cockpit. The Trakkabeam searchlight is also attached to the nose. Trakkabeams are used all over the world by airborne, ground and maritime law enforcement, as well as security, search and rescue, and medical emergency services. The centre fuselage includes the passenger cabin, while the rear fuselage holds the fuel tank bay and baggage compartment. The tail unit and tail plane include the fairings and stabilisers. The cowlings above the fuselage complete the overall aerodynamic shape of the aircraft and enclose the engines and main gearbox.

Landing gear

Different landing gear configurations (either fixed or retractable) are available, depending on the role of the helicopter, and the large wheels enable the aircraft to operate on unprepared terrain. The high landing gear, together with reduced floor thickness, provides a high ground clearance, together with easy access to the cabin.

The wheeled tricycle landing gear system includes two main landing gear and one nose landing gear. The main landing gear legs are equipped with one wheel, while the nose landing gear is equipped with two wheels. The nose landing gear wheel assembly and the main landing gear wheel assembly provide a better footprint on the ground, allowing the AW169 to

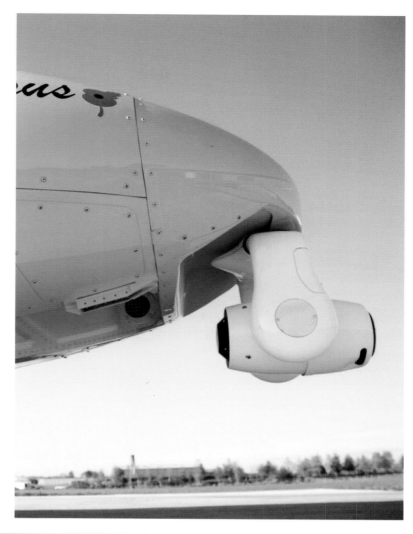

ABOVE The Trakkabeam searchlight is attached to the nose. *(Leonardo Helicopters/ Simon Pryor)*

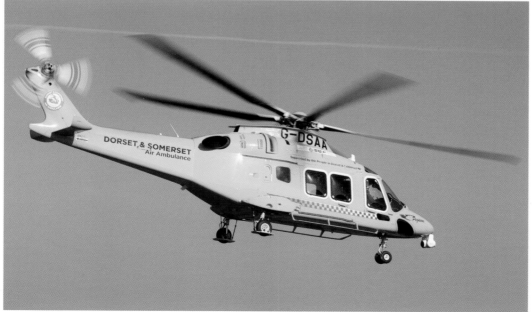

LEFT The wheeled tricycle landing gear system includes two main landing gear and one nose landing gear.

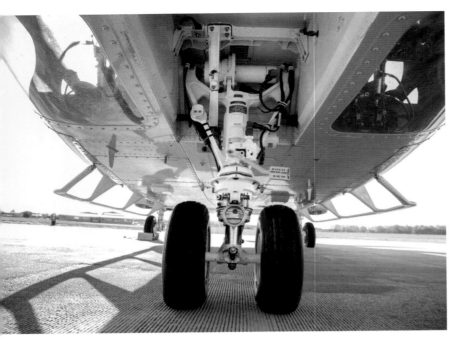

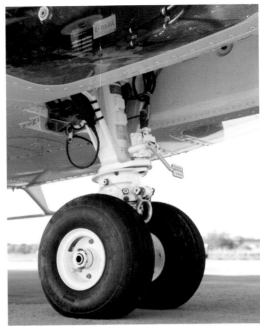

land in soft terrains without sinking. The landing gear is provided with hydraulic brakes on main wheels and the nose landing gear is equipped with an electrically operated centring lock.

The main landing gear is also fitted with so-called 'bear paws', which are pieces of equipment designed to prevent the aircraft from sinking into soft ground by spreading the weight of the helicopter over a much larger area than just the wheels. They are particularly beneficial for beach landings, as well as operations to fields, football pitches and parkland areas. Bear paws can be easily installed prior to the wet season and then removed for the summer months once the weather improves and the ground is consistently firmer.

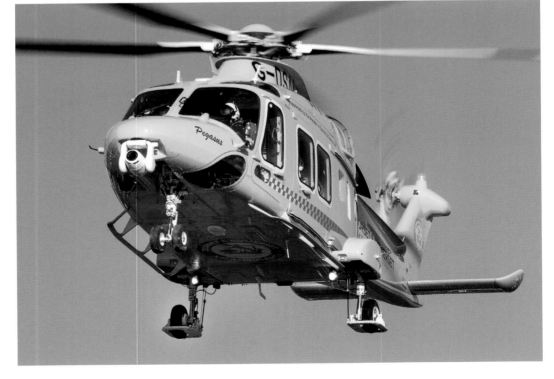

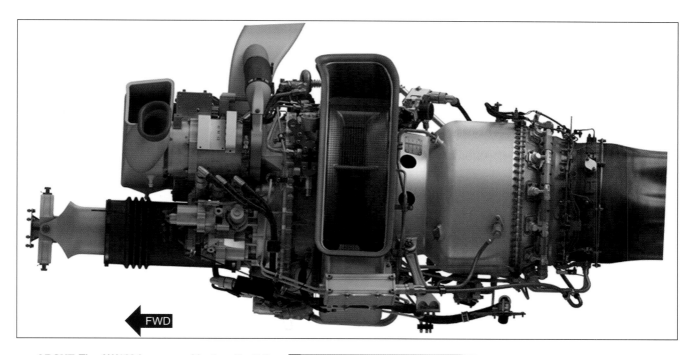

FWD

ABOVE The AW169 is powered by two Pratt & Whitney Canada PW210A turboshaft engines. The main output shaft can be seen bottom left, with the air intake duct for the compressor turbine in the centre. *(Leonardo Helicopters)*

RIGHT The AW169's compact PW210A engine installation (right-hand engine shown). *(Leonardo Helicopters)*

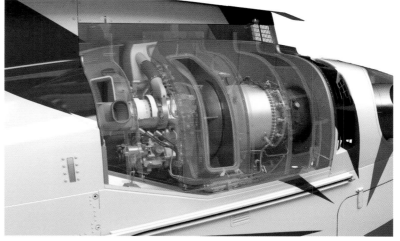

Engines

The power behind the AW169 is provided by two Pratt & Whitney Canada PW210A turboshaft engines. A turboshaft engine is essentially a jet engine, designed to drive a shaft. Whereas a conventional jet engine is designed to produce thrust, which propels the aircraft, the turboshaft engines in the AW169 drive both the main rotor via the main gearbox and the tail rotor via the main, intermediate and tail gearboxes. The engines also provide power for systems such as the avionics, via an accessory gearbox. In fact, on the PW210A engine, the accessory gearbox is integrated with the main reduction gearbox.

The PW210A incorporates the latest

RIGHT The right-hand engine on a winch being removed from DSAA's *Pegasus*, showing the compact packaging. *(Wayne Busby)*

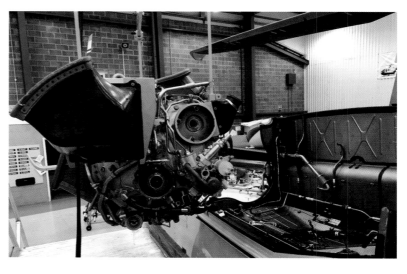

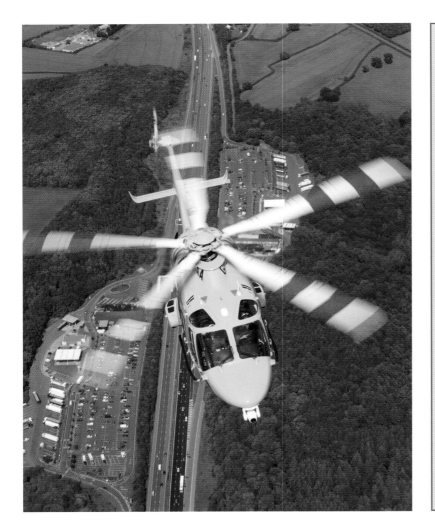

ABOVE Stripes painted on the rotor blades improve their visibility when rotating, both on the ground and airborne. *(Leonardo Helicopters/Simon Pryor)*

BELOW The AW169's main rotors have new fourth-generation blades, improving efficiency and reducing noise. *(Leonardo Helicopters)*

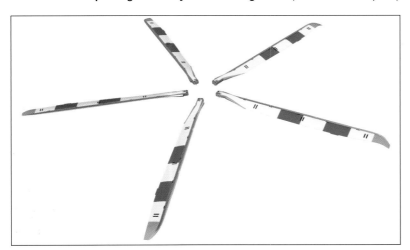

advances in compressor design technology and turbine materials. These advances give it an improved power-to-weight ratio, better fuel consumption, lower environmental emissions and better operating economics, all of which lead to an increased payload (the weight the helicopter can carry) and enhanced performance. The PW210A also incorporates a dual channel, Full Authority Digital Electronic Control (FADEC) system with state-of-the-art diagnostics capability, which controls all aspects of the engine's performance. The engines have been designed to fulfil the most stringent International Civil Aviation Organization industry emissions and noise standards, and include the most advanced environmental technologies.

Rotors

Helicopters are subject to substantial vibration and developments are constantly being made to help reduce this vibration and mitigate its effects. Elastomeric technology is one area that has helped to improve reliability – elastomeric components are made from bonded-rubber elastomeric elements, which are specially designed to eliminate certain types of vibration. The main rotor is a fully articulated system equipped with elastomeric bearings that allow the blades to flap, feather (change the angle), lead, lag and change pitch motions independently of each other. In a fully articulated system, each rotor blade is attached to the rotor hub through a series of hinges that lets each blade move independently of the others.

The main rotor is designed to deliver the power of the engine in the most efficient and effective way. The AW169 has new, fourth-generation main rotor blades, which means its efficiency in cruise flight (fast speed and low hourly fuel consumption) is combined with improved performance while hovering and at low speed. Inter-blade rotational dampers combine rubber and fluids to provide reduced vibrations and the design of this new generation of blades also significantly reduces the AW169's noise footprint.

The diameter of the main rotor is 12.12m (39ft 9in) and it is constructed using a combination of materials chosen for both their strength and their weight-saving properties. These include carbon and glass fibre composite materials, elastomeric bearing assemblies, titanium alloy, aluminium alloy and corrosion-resistant steel.

Incorrect assembly could result in the malfunction of the system, so each element of the hub and controls has been designed to avoid this. A wide range of elastomeric components have been used in order to reduce maintenance tasks, and with few parts to be checked, inspections are simpler and less frequent.

The AW169 tail rotor is a three-blade, fully articulated configuration, complete with new blade profiles, a rotor head with rotational elastomeric dampers (blade to hub) and all elastomeric bearings.

The high clearance of both rotors (main and tail) is an important feature for safe operations on the ground and in confined areas. The main rotor guarantees a clearance of 2.65m (8ft 8in) while the tail rotor, which is shielded by the tail

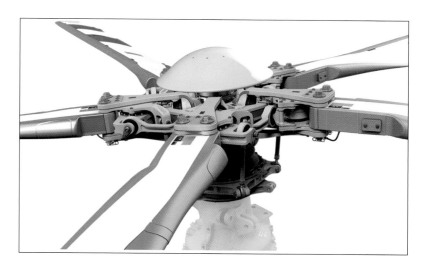

ABOVE AND BELOW Main rotor architecture, with inter-blade damper assembly shown below. *(Leonardo Helicopters)*

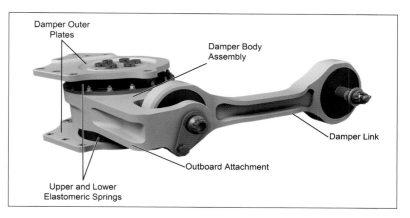

BELOW The AW169's tail rotor assembly. *(Leonardo Helicopters/Simon Pryor)*

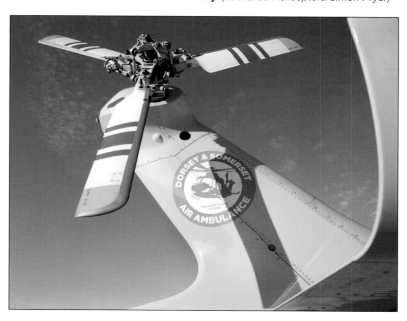

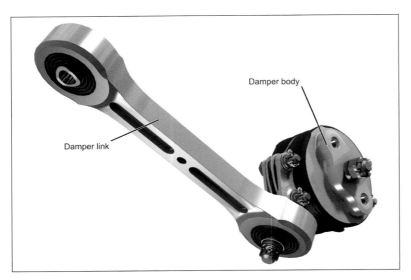

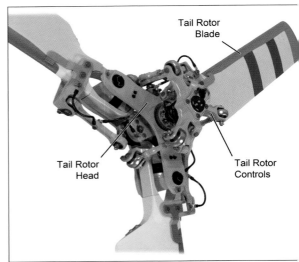

horizontal stabilisers, has a clearance of 2.16m (7ft 1in) , avoiding any unintentional contact with personnel working around the helicopter, particularly at night. This is particularly important for a service like the air ambulance, where the area around the helicopter could be accessed by people who are not trained to operate in a helicopter environment.

Transmission and Auxillary Power Unit (APU) mode

A helicopter's transmission system takes power from the engines and transmits it to the main and tail rotors. One of the purposes of the main gearbox is to reduce the output speed of the engine shaft from more than 20,000 rpm down to a few hundred rpm for the main rotor. The

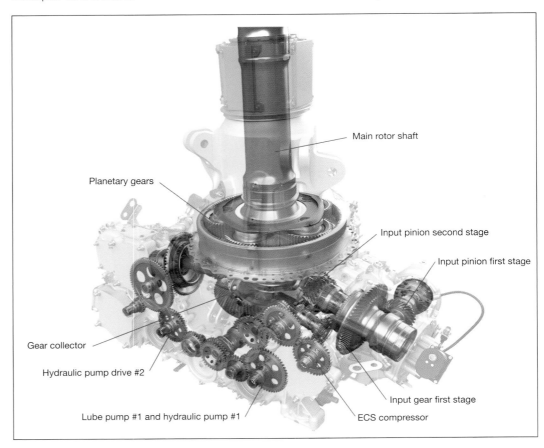

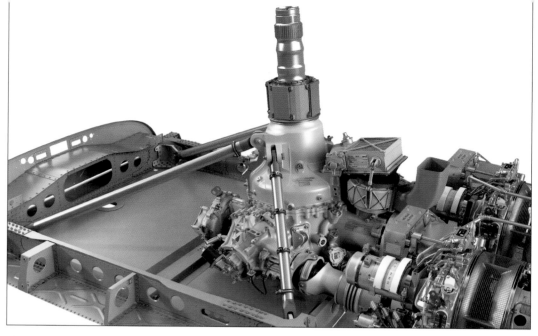

LEFT AW169 main gearbox installation, with PW210A engines visible to the right. *(Leonardo Helicopters)*

AW169's transmission design allows it to power the helicopter's systems even when the rotors are stopped. In order to achieve this, instead of having an APU, the AW169 has an APU mode integrated into the engine, meaning that access to all electrical capability is still available when the engine is running but the rotors have stopped.

The APU mode has a significant advantage when it comes to HEMS and patient transfer operations, as it gives the medical crew the chance to stabilise the patient in a controlled environment, away from rain, wind and external temperatures, before taking off. It also reduces noise and means there is no downwash (the air that is deflected by flowing around the rotors). This unique-in-its-class capability effectively transforms the AW169 into a flying operating room.

One slight disadvantage of the APU mode is that it takes fractionally longer to start up, because the two aircraft mission management computers need to talk to each other. However, a new software update will be available soon, which will remove those extra few seconds.

Air vehicle systems

The AW169 is an extremely complex aircraft, with dozens of systems working together to ensure its smooth, safe operation. Here is just a selection of some of the key systems:

Environmental Control System

The basic environmental control system consists of ventilation and heating, with air conditioning an optional extra. The ventilation system takes air from outside and ducts it through the cockpit and cabin areas to provide fresh air. The heating system takes bleed-air from the engines and mixes it with fresh air from outside to achieve the selected cockpit and cabin temperature. The heated air can also be directed to the cockpit windows to rapidly demist them. The system is designed to achieve

BELOW With the cowling off, the transmission can be seen here, with the output shaft from the right-hand engine arrowed. *(Wayne Busby)*

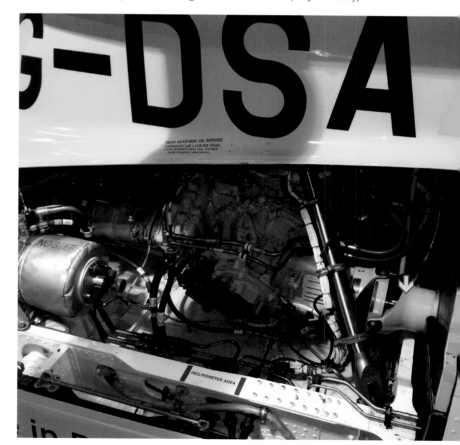

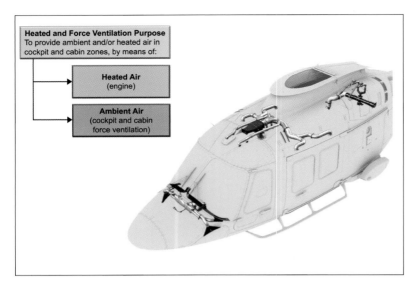

Heated and Force Ventilation Purpose
To provide ambient and/or heated air in cockpit and cabin zones, by means of:

- Heated Air (engine)
- Ambient Air (cockpit and cabin force ventilation)

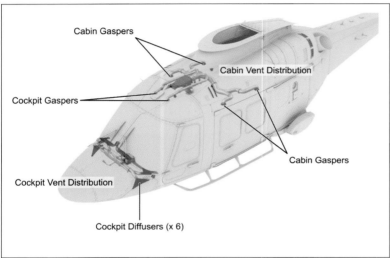

Cabin Gaspers

Cabin Vent Distribution

Cockpit Gaspers

Cabin Gaspers

Cockpit Vent Distribution

Cockpit Diffusers (x 6)

ABOVE AND BELOW Basic environmental control system (ECS) – vent distribution. *(Leonardo Helicopters)*

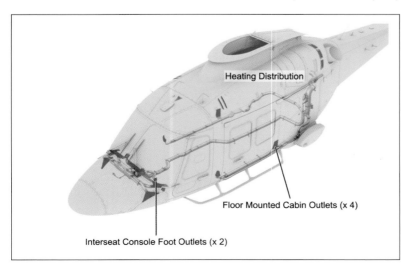

Heating Distribution

Floor Mounted Cabin Outlets (x 4)

Interseat Console Foot Outlets (x 2)

LEFT Basic environmental control system (ECS) – ventilation and heating. *(Leonardo Helicopters)*

at least +15°C (59°F) inside at the minimum aircraft operating temperature of -40°C (-40°F) outside. Cockpit ventilation air is distributed to two 'gaspers' (adjustable ventilation outlets) from the distribution device above the cabin roof. Further fresh air is provided from an intake at the front of the aircraft to six diffusers around the cockpit windows. Cabin fresh air is provided through four gaspers from above the cabin roof from the same distribution unit.

Fuel system

The fuel system provides fuel storage capability and supplies the two engines, at the pressure and flow rate requested by the engine, for aircraft operations in all ground and flight conditions. The basic system consists of two crash-resistant, interconnected cells. The fuel tanks are bladder type (essentially a rubberised bag) and have been manufactured and tested in order to meet the latest crash resistance requirements for flexible tank cells.

Hydraulic system

Rather like a power-assisted steering system on a car, the AW169's hydraulic system helps the pilot by reducing the amount of force needed to use the flying controls. The power control modules are installed on the upper deck in front of the main gearbox and they house most of the hydraulic system components, including the reservoir, shut-off valves, filters and sensors. The purpose of the power control modules is to store, filter and provide the hydraulic fluid, as well as monitor the pressure and temperature of the hydraulic system.

Electrical system

The main function of the electrical system is to provide electrical power to the helicopter systems and to start the engines. The electrical system in the AW169 is called the Electrical Power Generation and Distribution System (EPGDS). The EPGDS comprises all the equipment necessary to generate, convert and distribute electrical power around the helicopter.

Electrical power is fed into the power

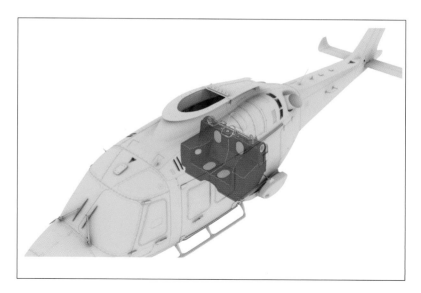

distribution units from the electrical power sources (starter generators, batteries and external power) and is then distributed via bus bars located in the circuit breaker panel and in the three remote electrical power units. Manual selection of power sources is possible from the EPGDS control panel and from the enhanced display control unit (EDCU). The two-touchscreen EDCUs are the main aircrew interface to control the electrical system.

Lighting

The basic aircraft is equipped with a complete package of lights to illuminate it both internally and externally to allow safe operational flying in all light conditions. The internal lighting system provides and manages illumination of the AW169's cockpit and cabin. Cockpit, cabin and baggage bay basic lights are night vision goggle (NVG) compatible, although the configuration of the cabin lights is dependent on the specific role of the AW169. Light emitting diode (LED) technology is widely used in order to reduce power consumption, maintenance operations and to provide increased reliability – no more bulbs to change. The main control panels for the cockpit lights system are the two EDCUs and the light control panel located in the interseat console. When the light control panel is switched to NIGHT mode position, all lights are automatically set to 20% brightness and the maximum level of display brightness available is reduced. The baggage compartment lights operate automatically through a microswitch on the baggage door.

The AW169's external lighting system is designed to meet requirements for both daylight and NVG operations. When the NVG kit is installed, the majority of the lighting subsystems can be operated in two modes; NORM (visible light source) and NVG (infrared light sources). The external lighting system provides external illumination, position identification and directional information to other aircraft and ground stations/operators. The basic external lighting system comprises steerable landing lights, position lights and anti-collision lights.

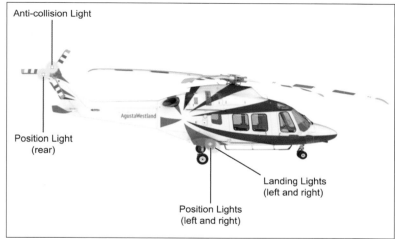

ABOVE AND BELOW **External light positions (above) and control screen (below).** *(Leonardo Helicopters)*

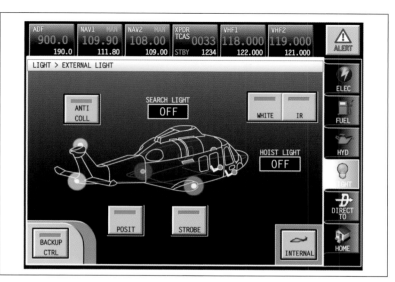

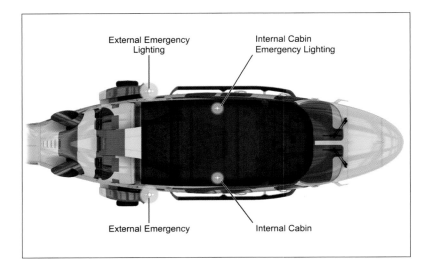

External Emergency
Lighting

Internal Cabin
Emergency Lighting

External Emergency

Internal Cabin

LEFT Emergency light locations.

(Leonardo Helicopters)

The aircraft is equipped with two identical steerable landing lights installed under the centre fuselage, inboard of the left and right main undercarriage, which assist with taxiing, take-offs and landings during night operations. The position lights and anti-collision lights are NVG-compatible light sources, using LED technology, and are positioned to avoid glare.

The emergency lights system comprises internal and external light sources to provide adequate light level in the event of an

NIGHT VISION GOGGLES

Night Vision Goggles (NVGs) look like a pair of ordinary binoculars and are worn in conjunction with a specially adapted helmet, which has a battery pack attached. Two image-intensifying tubes amplify the available light and project pictures onto the small screens inside the goggles. Traditionally, NVGs have a green display but DSAA's NVGs have a black-and-white display, which is even sharper.

NVGs enable pilots to see what is going on outside, even in almost complete darkness. They focus and adjust automatically and are mounted an inch or so away from the eyes, so the pilot is able to look beneath them and see the instrument panel. The helicopter cockpit has to have specially adapted blue/green lights on the instrument panel so that these lights don't affect the goggles and a curtain between cockpit and cabin prevents the goggles from being affected by other light that may be present in the cabin.

Flying with goggles allows the pilot to see other aircraft, roads, rivers and railways, which helps with navigation and they also

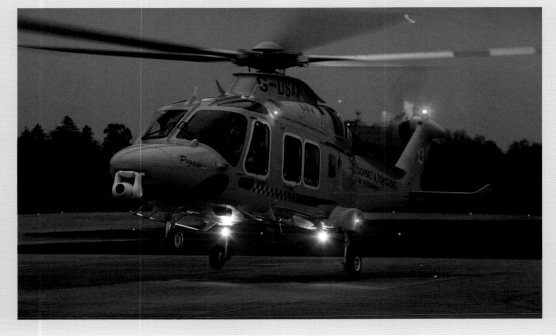

RIGHT Now that DSAA undertakes night HEMS, the latest night-vision technology is provided to assist the crew.

emergency landing with loss of the aircraft electrical generation and power distribution system. All components and wiring are physically and electrically segregated from the normal system. An emergency battery pack provides power for the required level of illumination for at least 20 minutes after an emergency landing or failure. Two internal emergency lights are installed above the centre of each sliding door to provide illumination of the passenger exits within the cabin. The two external emergency lights use LED technology to produce white light that illuminates the terrain around the AW169's exits in the event of an emergency landing.

Avionics

Avionics are the electronic devices and systems in an aircraft, and the AW169 contains extremely advanced technology. The cutting-edge avionics suite includes an electronic flight instrument system, dual flight management system, state-of-the-art navigation system, and digital autopilot and helicopter terrain awareness warning system, all of which help to reduce the workload of the crew.

Integrated into the avionics is an aircraft mission management system, which helps to operate the helicopter. This digital system monitors and controls operations and is comprised of two aircraft and mission

give a great view of the horizon, which helps with orientation. In a HEMS operation, the pilot can see the landing site much earlier, so can plan their approach. It also helps the medical crew, as they wear the goggles too, allowing them to orientate themselves on the scene rather than struggling in the darkness. NVGs can't detect some hard-to-see obstacles, such as telegraph wires, for example. This is countered by rigorous flight planning to assess the terrain, with the crew amassing as much data as possible before they take off.

There needs to be some background light for NVGs to work, whether starlight, moonlight or 'cultural' light, which is light from streetlamps, houses or from the helicopter itself. Bright lights, such as car headlights or torches shone directly towards them can be a problem – but if the wearer looks at a bright light while wearing NVGs, the goggles will instantly adjust by reducing the gain on that area.

When it comes to weather, NVGs enable the pilot to see through haze and mist, which could potentially lead them to fly on into decreasing visibility, meaning a back-up plan is necessary if the aircraft should end up in a cloud, for example. NVGs also provide a reduced field of vision and no 3D vision, so gauging distances of objects using other cues is vital. They are also heavy and a little cumbersome, so wearing them is itself a skill.

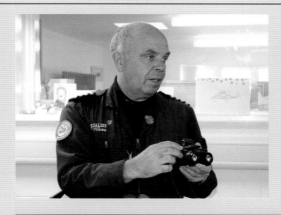

LEFT Unit Chief Pilot Mario Carretta briefing his team on use of NVGs.

BELOW NVGs enable the crew members to see what is going on outside, even in almost complete darkness.

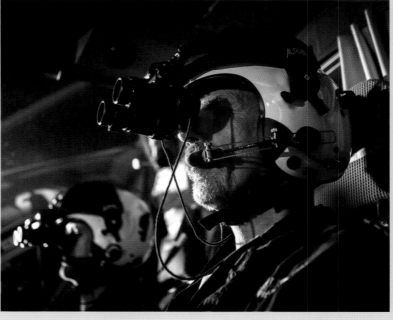

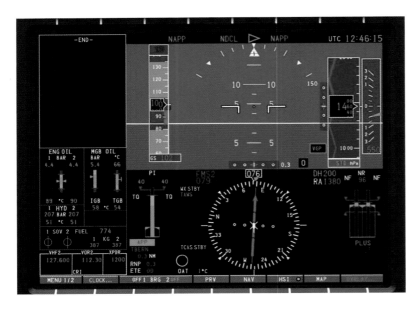

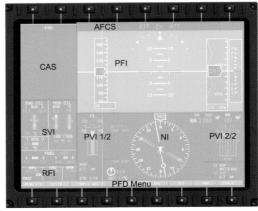

LEFT AND ABOVE Primary flight display basic layout. *(Leonardo Helicopters)*

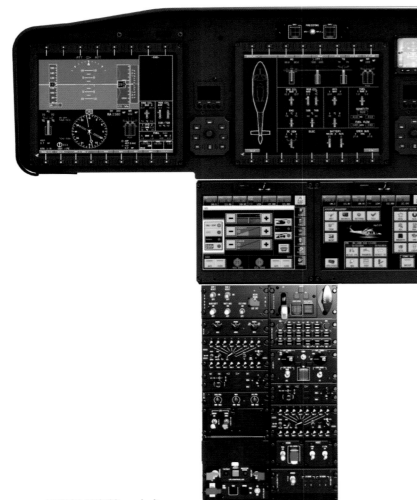

RIGHT AW169 cockpit controls layout.
(Leonardo Helicopters)

management computers, two touch-screen enhanced display and control units and one data transfer device. At the core of this integrated platform is a high-speed digital bus. In avionics terms, a bus (a contraction of the Latin 'omnibus') is a communication system that transfers data between components inside a computer or between multiple computers. The AW169's bus connects the cockpit displays, the main computers and the enhanced display and control units.

Cockpit display system

The cockpit display system is based on three 10 x 8in (25 x 20cm), landscape orientated, active-matrix liquid-crystal displays, two primary flight displays and one multi-function display. The landscape orientation of the displays optimises the visualisation of electro-optical and infrared sensors, maps and external camera image output. The system is designed for single/dual pilot operation.

The primary flight display shows the primary attitude (orientation of the helicopter relative to the horizon), heading, altitude, airspeed, navigation and flight guidance functions, as well as displaying messages from the crew-alerting system, primary engine data and radio tuning frequencies. The AW169's primary flight display layout has been designed using the 'Common Cockpit Concept' approach, which means it shares the same avionics layout displays and AgustaWestland proprietary software with the AW189 and the same avionic system set-up as the AW139. This layout was designed to provide pilots with operational and training advantages when switching from one helicopter type to the other.

The multi-function display is a multi-windowed display that can be configured with a variety of layout and pages, including power plant pages, synoptic displays, maintenance information and video display. There are also two identical display control panels located in the cockpit, on the forward edges of the interseat console, which allow the pilot to manage some parameters on a display unit.

Automatic Flight Control System

The AW169 has a four-axis digital Automatic Flight Control System (AFCS). The AFCS provides stability and control augmentation functions, self-test, monitoring functions and flight director modes. The auto-stabilisation part of the system provides short-term corrections against unwanted events such as turbulence, making for a smoother flight, while the autopilot part of the AFCS carries out long-term corrections. The AFCS is also coupled through the flight management system to the navigation systems. The AFCS performs its functions based on the processing capabilities provided by the flight control computer (FCC). The FCC has two independent channels (designated channel 1 and channel 2) and each channel is powered by an independent power supply unit.

Navigation system

The navigation system allows the pilot to determine the position and direction of the aircraft on or above the surface of the Earth. The navigation system supplies the aircraft navigation

BELOW The cockpit display system is based on three 10 x 8in (25 x 20cm), landscape-orientated, active-matrix liquid-crystal displays.

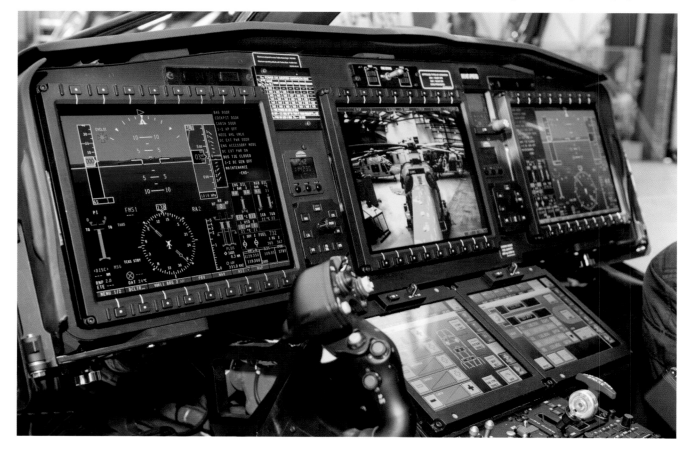

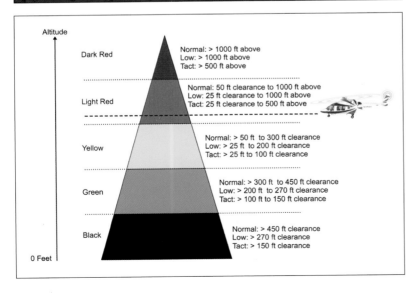

LEFT Synthetic vision display. *(Leonardo Helicopters)*

data in order to provide flight planning capability, navigation information and flight performance data to pilot and co-pilot. It includes the following sub-systems: flight environment data; attitude and direction; landing aid system; radio altimeter system; position determining system; and flight management system.

Flight Environment Data

The flight environment data system uses sensors to measure the different environmental conditions, such as air pressure, airspeed, altitude and outside air temperature.

Synthetic Vision System

When the air ambulance is called out in adverse weather conditions, in poor visibility or even at night, the synthetic vision system proves very useful. By using data from obstacle, terrain and other databases to generate a virtual landscape, the system can provide a digital view of the outside world, leading to improved flight safety at the most critical phases of a mission, such as landing or taking off.

Helicopter Terrain Awareness Warning Ssystem

The helicopter terrain awareness warning system does what it says on the tin: providing the pilot with information on surrounding terrain and obstacles that may pose a collision risk, using a colour-coded display.

Flight Management System

The Fight Management System (FMS) provides flight planning capability, navigation information and flight performance data, managing flight details from take-off to touchdown. It provides detailed predictions regarding the estimated time and fuel remaining along the entire flight plan and, using this information, can perform accurate, long-range, lateral and vertical navigation. The pilot controls the FMS operations via the touch-screen displays, while the active flight plan information is displayed on the multi-function display.

CENTRE AND LEFT HTAWS display details.

(Leonardo Helicopters)

Communications system

The communications system provides routing and control of all internal and external communications. The system also integrates audio from the crew-alerting system (CAS) and radio navigation aids. The interphone communication system provides the control and routing for all internal communications between the crew in the cockpit and in the cabin, as well as radio and navigation audio-only sources. An external intercom socket allows ground crew to connect a headset, enabling them to talk to the crew over the aircraft intercom.

External communication takes place using the VHF communication system, with two VHF amplitude modulation (AM) transceivers (VHF 1 and VHF 2), each connected to a dedicated antenna.

Indicating and Recording System

The indicating and recording system is the means by which voice and flight data is recorded.

The cockpit and voice flight data recording system has an underwater locator beacon that will transmit for a period of 30 days and can operate to a depth of 20,000ft (6,100m). The main recording unit retains the last 25 hours of aircraft data and the most recent two hours of cockpit audio sources. The data is stored in a crash survivable memory module to enable retrieval and decoding for analysis, should an accident occur. In that event, an emergency

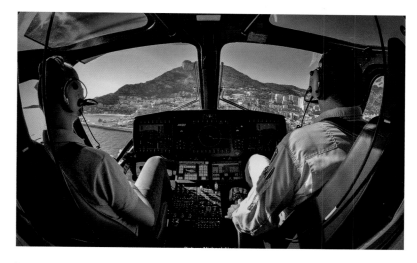

locator transmitter will automatically activate and send an encoded digital message containing the aircraft's serial number and its last position.

Cockpit

The forward section of the fuselage contains the fully digital 'glass' cockpit, which holds the instrument panels and all the pilot and co-pilot controls. The cockpit combines the latest avionics with extremely good external visibility, which maximises situational awareness and reduces pilot workload to increase operational safety. It features an ice and rain protection system and a windshield wiping system that keeps the windshield surface clean from water, dirt, sand, dust or a thin coating of soft snow.

The cockpit has forward-opening hinged

ABOVE The cockpit's outstanding external visibility is particularly effective during take-off/landing procedures. *(Leonardo Helicopters)*

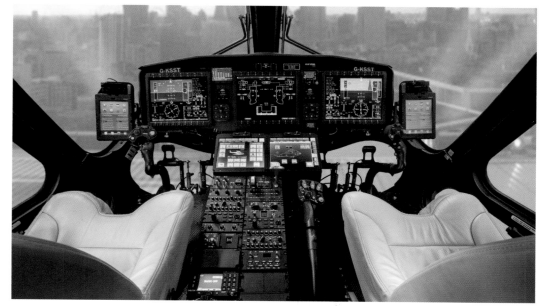

LEFT The cockpit combines the latest avionics with generous internal dimensions. *(Leonardo Helicopters/ Simon Pryor)*

doors (with a storm window on the pilot's side), and steps for cockpit entry. Pilot and co-pilot doors are provided with pop-out windows that ensure a quick evacuation of the helicopter in case of emergency. The generous internal dimensions of the cockpit ($3m^3$/$106ft^3$) provide a large workspace for the pilots. The pilot and co-pilot have adjustable crashworthy seats with safety harnesses.

Cabin

The cabin is where most of the bespoke HEMS features can be found. Senior DSAA clinicians worked closely with Specialist Aviation Services (SAS) to design a future-proof cabin, so the team could change how it operates down the line without making significant alterations to the aircraft. The key considerations were how they might carry a patient and what equipment they needed to take with them.

Centralising the patient had proved impossible on any previous airframe, as none were wide enough. Even the larger airframes on the market don't provide access to both sides of the patient, meaning the treatment a

patient could receive in transit was restricted, as clinicians in the back could only really access patients from the waist up, rather than access the patient's whole body.

In this configuration, the AW169's cabin provides full access to the patient's entire body from top to toe, including access to both sides, as well as providing a spacious and bright working environment for the medical crew. The patient is placed in a central, comfortable position, with optimal height and natural light, surrounded by the clinical team.

DSAA also explored how the team could access the patient more effectively while remaining strapped in, so it worked with SAS to develop a rotating seat, which can slide out next to the patient and move up and down alongside them.

Its flat floor and ceiling design mean that the cabin also provides plenty of space ($6.3m^3$/$222ft^3$), with a total width of 2.03m (6ft 1in) and constant height of 1.32m (4ft 4in). With such a large cabin, the AW169 can accommodate a variety of internal layouts and this gave the DSAA plenty of flexibility when it came to configuration.

BELOW The AW169's larger cabin area gives full access to the patient.

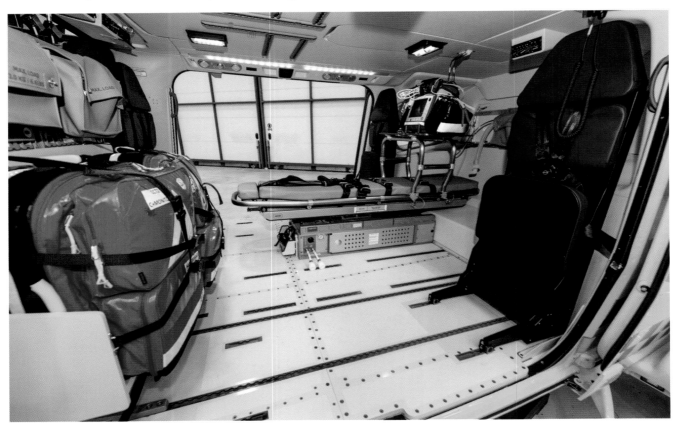

The cabin needed to be as clutter-free as possible, particularly the headspace. In the AW169 nothing is hanging off the roof. When treating a patient, the crew members can't walk around, they need to crouch, so having things hanging from the roof restricts their movement. The box-shaped interior is unique. Where other aircraft ceilings slope down, the headspace is very restricted and comes too close to the patient for the clinician to have much movement, meaning a very limited environment for continued resuscitation. Phil Hyde, DSAA Medical Lead, explained that the team used to prefer to take a patient to hospital by road just because of this issue of limited space. This new working environment has opened up new possibilities of providing care en route, which he describes as a game changer.

There's also much more space to store things in the AW169. In the EC135, the Scoop (yellow rescue stretcher) had to sit on the litter, with the crew's kit bags on top of it. The bags were all strapped on and needed unstrapping on arrival, all of which took precious seconds. Rather than cluttering the cabin with drawers or cupboards, the AW169 has purpose-designed storage compartments where the kit bags can be placed and the crew simply unclip them and get away cleanly and quickly. A spacious baggage compartment provides an additional 1.4m³ (50ft³) of separate space to stow loose equipment and can sustain a load of up to 250kg (550lb), which helps to keep the crew's working environment uncluttered.

The adjustable seats can be quickly removed if necessary and each comes with a four-point seatbelt. The seats are equipped with an energy absorbing system, which reduces crash impact by transferring the load to the aircraft structure, thus increasing chances of survivability in the event of a crash.

Integrated oxygen and electrical system outlets are provided all around the cabin, while the ceiling is equipped with patient lights, tracks for medical equipment and safety hooks.

The cabin is accessible through two wide sliding doors, one on each side of the helicopter, measuring 1.6m (5ft 3in) wide and 1.2m (3ft 11in) high. These give fast and complete access to the whole cabin from both sides of the helicopter. The helicopter's belly clearance from the ground is 0.5m (1ft 8in) while the cabin doors' sill height is 0.65m (2ft 2in), which provides enough external obstacle clearance while still allowing passengers to easily access the cabin.

The patient loading system houses the oxygen system and makes it easy to move patients into the aircraft. It incorporates a detachable stretcher unit, which is secured directly to the base with a single locking mechanism, without the need for additional belts or harnesses. It also includes a backrest section that can be raised in all phases of flight, to enable flexible positioning of the patient to optimise care during transportation. The stretcher itself is 195cm (6ft 5in) long and its surface is made up of closed cell foam pads, upholstered with a tough, non-absorbent, antibacterial material.

All monitoring and electronic equipment that supports the patient, including drug infusing pumps and ventilators, are placed around the patient, rather than hanging off them. This saves having wires and tubes hanging freely, or crew members having to hold lines or place equipment on top of the patient. In older aircraft, patients who were intubated

BELOW The baggage compartment provides an additional 1.4m³ (50ft³) of separate space to stow loose equipment.

BOTTOM The adjustable seats can be quickly removed if necessary and are equipped with an energy absorbing system, to reduce impact in the event of a crash. *(Leonardo Helicopters)*

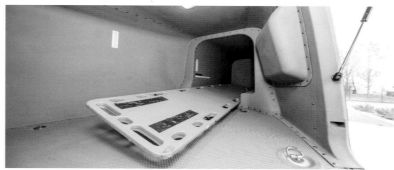

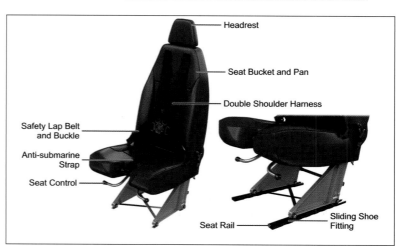

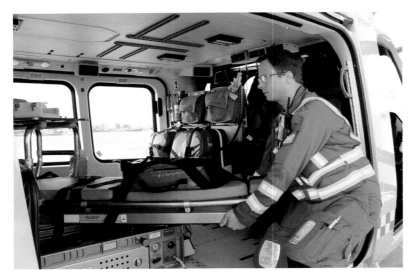

ABOVE The bespoke patient loading system rotates through 90° and makes it easy to move patients in and out of the aircraft, with a detachable stretcher assembly.

BELOW Working with DSAA, Specialist Aviation Services (SAS) came up with an initial concept for the cabin design (the Trakkabeam searchlight mounting is shown here). *(SAS)*

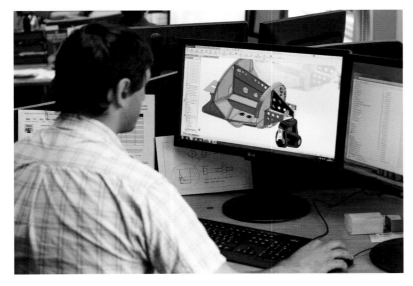

had to be pushed through the boot of the aircraft, meaning the patient would have to be disconnected from life support and swiftly reconnected if they were moved by air. This is life-sustaining equipment and when patients are being moved, there is always a danger that lines will be pulled out.

To address this, DSAA asked SAS to create a bespoke stretcher bridge that sits across the patient and upon which the monitoring equipment, ventilators and drug infusion pumps are placed, all centralised within the linear construct of the stretcher. The bridge is used on scene, then it can transition into the aircraft and later into the hospital, if necessary. The patient is therefore packaged cleanly, vital lines cannot be pulled out while they are being moved, and the hospital staff who receive them know where

to find all the equipment on the patient's body. Other air ambulances have now adopted this type of bridge in their aircraft.

The service has now brought another layer of monitoring capability into the aircraft, measuring blood pressure directly from the arteries of the patient. Having a simple, operational and elegant design right from the beginning means that DSAA is able to constantly improve how much its clinicians can do for patients.

Designing for HEMS operations

Specialist Aviation Services (SAS) was responsible for customising the AW169 for HEMS operations with DSAA under the watchful eye of Jan-Marc van Dam, the company's director of completions, head of design and chief of office of airworthiness. This involved design and installation of the nose-mounted searchlight, tactical radios and, of course, the HEMS interior. SAS was one of the launch customers for the AW169 and is the world's largest operator of the type, so the company enjoys a close working relationship with Leonardo Helicopters.

During the standard design process, the customer comes up with a spec or wish list, which is discussed with SAS's designers before work starts on an initial concept. This is an iterative process, with the client and designer going backwards and forwards until they get the concept more or less right. The project then moves on to a more detailed design process and, parallel to that, the certification and manufacturing processes begin.

For a HEMS interior, it is actually quite difficult for the client to write a detailed specification or definitive set of requirements; most people have a clear idea in their minds of what they want, but find that putting that on paper, in terms equally understood by aerospace engineers and medical specialists, a challenge. 'On the other hand, you can over-design something,' says Jan-Marc. 'Because the AW169 was such a step change from the existing aircraft, it was important not to over-analyse it, but to get it into service initially and then, as experience is gained, adapt the interior and operating procedures to suit.'

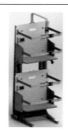

- Initial proposal to have two shelves on a single rack based upon an existing design.
- Customer request to retain existing kit bags and dimensions.
- Design modified to match customer request at the loss of a seating position.
- Space made available for optional additional storage or equipment.

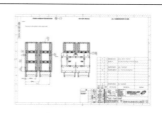

LEFT Work sheets showing the iterative design process for various aspects of the AW169's HEMS interior. *(SAS)*

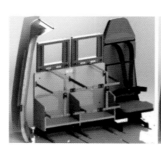

- Customer requested the facility to carry, and use in-flight, two (2) Fresnius Kabi Injectomat syringe drivers.
- The shape and functionality of the hardware limited possible installation positions within the aircraft utilising free space.
- Limited access to the syringe driver meant creating a simple concept of a retention mount.
- Loan of actual hardware allowed for a detailed survey of the equipment and the creation of an accurate space model of the syringe driver.
- A more suitable retention method created to better suit the complex shape of the syringe driver and allowed for adjustment.

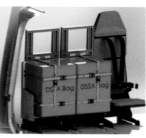

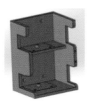

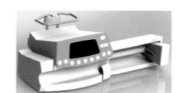

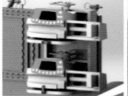

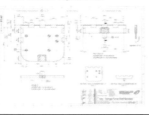

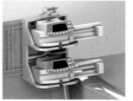

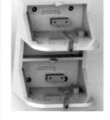

- Customer requested a fixed stretcher bridge.
- Design limited by available space within the cabin and strength of mounting components.
- Equipment to be carried was not fully decided.
- Removable shelf and lightweight bridge requested for ground carrying to/from incidents with common interfaces.
- Customer created a mock-up based upon dimensions provided. To check feasibility

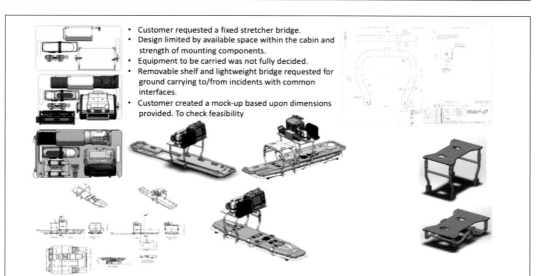

The baseline medical interior for the AW169 was designed in close co-operation with Kent, Surrey and Sussex Air Ambulance's medical team. There are eight people in the Staverton design team, plus Jan-Marc; typically, one designer is assigned as a point of contact and sits down with the client's senior clinicians and literally asks: 'What would you like?' Flexibility and future-proofing is an important part of the process. If an aircraft is designed around an organisation's current way of operating, there is a danger that the organisation will just end up with another version of what it already has. A better starting point is to consider how you would like to operate and then design around that.

As we have mentioned, the unique positioning of the stretcher is key for SAS's HEMS customers. The factory fit of an Emergency Medical Services AW169 interior has a sideways stretcher, which is fine for mountain rescue but not for an air ambulance. 'This would have been a show stopper,' explains Jan-Marc. 'The patient had to be placed longitudinally in the cabin – if that couldn't be done, the medical teams didn't want the aircraft.'

The main reason for this placement is airway management. A patient suffering from trauma, who might be anaesthetised, can get sick very quickly and the clinical team need to have someone at the head of the patient to unblock their airway rapidly. In *Pegasus*, the patient is just off-centre to the right, which has added benefits while loading. The patient is loaded from the right-hand side of the aircraft because the pilot sits on the right and so can watch the loading occur. Also, unique to the AW169, the APU mode means an engine can be left running without the rotors turning, providing electrical power, light and air conditioning. On the AW169, this is the left-hand engine, so that side of the aircraft is much noisier and you would obviously want to load the patient on the side with less noise. By having the stretcher slightly off-centre, the clinicians also don't have to reach as far into the cabin to load the patient. When dealing with a heavy patient or lots of equipment, multiple people are needed to load the aircraft and having the stretcher offset to the right makes this easier.

DSAA was the third air ambulance to take on an AW169, after Kent, Surrey and Sussex Air Ambulance and Lincolnshire & Nottinghamshire Air Ambulance, although the first to be in operational service. The DSAA team was able to look at the choices their colleagues at other units had made, then add their own specific requirements. SAS came up with an initial 3D computer-aided design (CAD) concept and then discussed with DSAA the changes that needed to be made.

For SAS, the three principal contacts at DSAA were Phil Hyde (Medical Lead), Paul Owen (Operational Lead) and Owen Hammett (Critical Care Practitioner). Owen's background as a medical device technician was particularly helpful because he understood how the different devices could be taken apart and knew what might be likely to break. Designing a complex interior like this would have been very difficult by committee, as too many different opinions would have greatly slowed the project down. Jan-Marc found the experience of working with the trio from DSAA very positive as they worked extremely effectively together. 'The fascinating thing was that we rarely had all three contacts at the same meeting, but they all knew exactly what the others wanted and would agree to,' explains Jan-Marc. 'They did a brilliant job of synchronising their views and communicating between themselves. If you said something to Paul on one day and met Phil the next day, he would be aware of it.'

DSAA took a very pragmatic approach to this, using the CAD concept to create what Jan-Marc refers to as a '*Blue Peter*' mock-up – their own physical version of a cabin using wood, cardboard and canteen chairs to see how the team would be able to operate in the space. While the CAD drawings are very detailed, they are just a representation of reality and the team found that creating a physical design that they could actually try out helped them to see whether they could reach things comfortably and work effectively in the space. Some detailed changes were made because of that simulation and instead of the design being merely adequate, it ended up being exactly what the team wanted.

Using the feedback gained so far, the interior concept was refined until it was signed off. A preliminary design review was held, where the initial concept was shown and all the requirements were discussed and nailed down. The concept is then

SAS: SPECIALIST AVIATION SERVICES

Specialist Aviation Services (SAS) Group was created some 30 years ago, during the infancy of emergency services aviation. SAS was initially called Police Aviation Services (PAS), as its origins were in the provision of helicopters for the police service. However, as demand for emergency medical aviation services grew, dedicated aeromedical aircraft began to emerge and so PAS created Medical Aviation Services (MAS) to operate in that market. SAS, as the company is now known, is privately owned and operates MD 902 and AW169 helicopters.

In recent years, the police side of the business has taken a back seat. While SAS still provides maintenance support for the police forces of Belgium, Luxembourg and Kuwait, it no longer does any police-related work in the UK. Instead, HEMS has become SAS's core business, with the company now having about 40% of the UK HEMS market. It has become a pioneer in the field with the operation of the AW169, which has provided a step change in capability for the UK's air ambulance services.

SAS offers completion, role-equipping and modification of aircraft used for emergency services and other applications. It has a comprehensive in-house design and manufacturing capability and can install mission management systems for police aircraft, medical interiors for air ambulances and load-lifting equipment for offshore helicopters. Working closely with specialist equipment suppliers, SAS can integrate its equipment into customers' aircraft as well as designing brand-new modifications in-house. The company's design philosophy is to create aircraft that are fit for purpose, easy to maintain and easy to adapt, as well as meeting all health and safety and certification requirements. It can provide a comprehensive 24/7 support capability and has a strategic spares and logistics operation. Aircraft interiors can be reconfigured quickly and cheaply to keep up with changes to the medical equipment or even developments in operational thinking.

SAS also recruits, trains and provides the pilots to fly its AW169s and MD 902s. Pilots travel to Leonardo's training facility in Italy to undergo training and receive their type rating before returning to the UK to be dispatched to a unit. Some pilots work full time with a particular HEMS and some are floating pilots, covering gaps when other pilots are unavailable, on holiday or in training.

While some SAS clients own their aircraft and just use SAS to provide maintenance, the contract with DSAA means SAS provides the full service: the aircraft, all of the airworthiness associated with it, the engineers, the maintenance and the pilots. SAS is not a particularly large corporate entity so it can flex around a customer's demands.

Adaptations and improvements can be undertaken during the course of any leasing contract. One example of this with DSAA was the introduction of night vision capability, which requires modifications to the aircraft, changes to crew shift patterns and training in the use of night vision goggles.

SAS engineers and designers worked closely with DSAA to guide the charity through the practical aspects of what needed to be achieved in order to secure clearance to operate. The combined efforts of the two organisations mean that patients can now be treated in-flight in a way they never could have previously.

The company has 170 employees, including 60 pilots and 50 engineers. Its headquarters can be found at Gloucestershire Airport in England and it also has a facility at Redhill near Gatwick, England and in Genk, Belgium.

BELOW DSAA's pilots and engineers are all recruited, trained and employed by Specialist Aviation Services (SAS), the operator of its AW169 air ambulance.

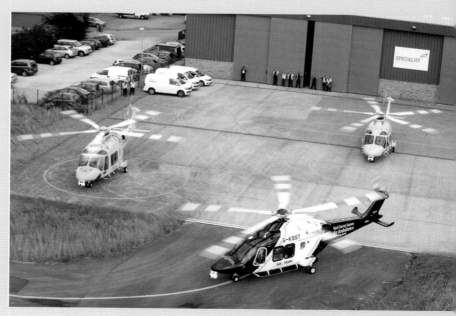

developed further and improved upon before the critical design review (CDR) is held. Once the CDR has been completed there should be no further changes. After this point, drawings get released and parts get made – or, in Jan-Marc's words: 'We are cutting metal.' If changes are made after this, it isn't necessarily a problem, but SAS would no longer be able to guarantee the changes would be incorporated before the planned entry into service date.

In a project as demanding and complex as this, ongoing consultation and communication throughout the whole process is vital. 'You don't just meet each other once or twice and then never discuss things again,' says Jan-Marc. Having a close and productive working relationship is key: 'These are all long-term contracts,' he says. 'You are dealing with people for seven to ten years, so there is no point in falling out over what is just a minor change.'

Flexibility is important, as circumstances can change at any point, making it necessary to alter things at different stages in the process. *Pegasus* had a last-minute change to its design because DSAA wanted to use a new type of vital signs monitor; that particular monitor wasn't ready in the configuration desired, so they had to go back to the original monitor, meaning a change to the design was needed. For SAS, one advantage of creating their own interiors is that they can easily adapt them without having to involve a third party.

SAS does some of the manufacturing in-house, while some is outsourced to specialist aircraft interior manufacturing companies. The basic construction techniques are very similar to those you would find in an airline galley. Once the parts have been manufactured, they are installed and tested and the aircraft can be released for service.

Parallel to the manufacturing runs the process of certification. Because the AW169 is a civil-registered aircraft operating under UK air transport rules, it must be certified in accordance with European Aviation Safety Agency (EASA) regulations. When it comes to modifications, there are so-called minor and major changes. Minor changes are modifications that SAS can authorise and approve itself, while major changes must go back to EASA for approval. Because of the

extent of the modifications in *Pegasus*, this was classed as a major change and thus the extended approval process had to happen.

During the certification process, SAS must demonstrate to the authority that the modification meets the airworthiness specifications. CAD-renderings of the interior and isometric views of components allow SAS to brief the authority on what the aircraft will look like.

SAS has to compile a number of compliance demonstration reports, including the stress reports, as well as looking at other potential issues, such as whether any of the materials were flammable. Some of those reports are submitted to the authority and may result in further discussions. In particular, the oxygen system had to comply with the latest EASA rules in order to be certified and that took longer than anticipated.

Once all compliance reports have been completed, all EASA queries have been resolved and the compliance checklist is complete, SAS submits a Declaration of Compliance to EASA. If EASA agrees, it will issue the Supplemental Type Certificate (STC) for the emergency medical services interior. Once the STC has been issued, the parts can be approved and issued with an EASA Form 1, showing that they not only conform to the drawing but they are also safe, approved and can be installed on any in-service aircraft. At that point, the aircraft can also be put into service.

'Across our fleet we work with four different vital signs monitors, six different ventilators and three different oxygen bottles,' explains Jan-Marc. 'You need to keep the interior modular so you can adjust it to whatever that customer or road ambulance region uses.' The UK's different regional ambulance services work in different ways and use different equipment: oxygen bottles, for example, need to match those that the local ambulance service uses, so the AW169 needs to be able to carry the correct equipment rather than having incompatible oxygen systems.

Jan-Marc describes the concept behind the interior as being like Lego bricks, with the backbone being the main STC. The STC means the interior is already approved by EASA, with a number of seating arrangements, and then SAS can adjust things like shelves, cabinets or the stretcher bridge around this backbone, depending on what works for a particular customer.

Assembly

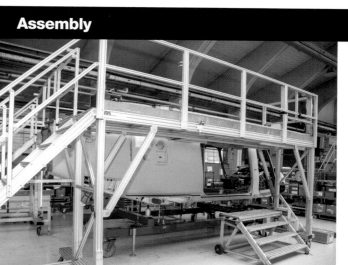

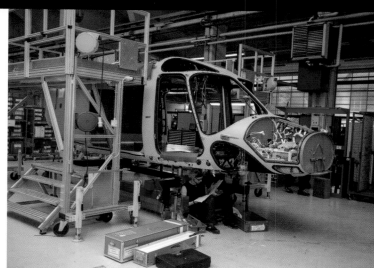

ABOVE An AW169 near the start of the final assembly process at Leonardo Helicopters' Vergiate facility in Northern Italy. The tail structure will be bolted on later. *(Leonardo Helicopters)*

ABOVE RIGHT Here wiring looms are being installed into the airframe. *(Leonardo Helicopters)*

RIGHT Here further wiring looms, the cockpit display panel and avionics are being installed. *(Leonardo Helicopters)*

BELOW RIGHT Here the engine, main gearbox and tail rotor have been installed. *(Leonardo Helicopters)*

BELOW This shows the cockpit display panel and flying controls in position. *(Leonardo Helicopters)*

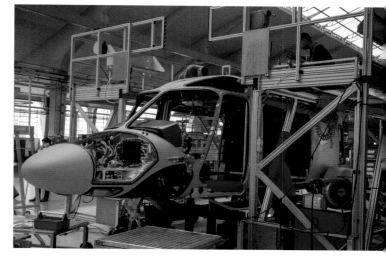

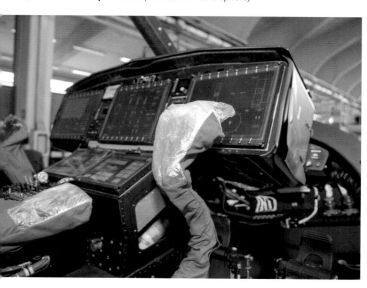

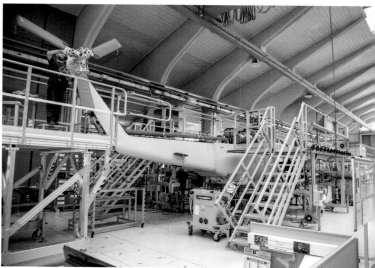

CHARACTERISTICS

Dual or Single Pilot Configuration

Minimum operating temperature	-40°C	
Maximum operating temperature	50°C (or ISA +35)	
Flight envelope	up to 15,000ft	
Take-off and landings	up to 15,000ft HD	
Maximum speed	@5,000ft	153 ktas
Recommended cruise speed	@5,000ft	135 ktas
Maximum rate of climb	1,847ft/min	9.38m/s
Range (at recommended cruise speed 5,000ft)	446nm	826km
Endurance (at best endurance speed, 5,000ft)	4hrs 23 mins	
Maximum take-off weight	4,600/4,800kg	10,141/10,582lb
Cabin volume (single pilot)	7.5m^3	265ft^3
Max gross weight	4,600/4,800kg	10,141/10,582lb
Propulsion	2 x Pratt & Whitney Canada PW210A series turboshafts with FADEC	

External Dimensions

Overall length*	14.65m	48ft 01in
Overall height*	4.50m	14ft 09in
Rotor diameter	12.12m	39ft 09in

Internal Dimensions: Cockpit

Max length	1.62m	5ft 4in
Max width	2.15m	7ft 1in
Max height	1.42m	4ft 8in

Internal Dimensions: Cabin

Length	2.15m	7ft 1in
Max width	2.03m	6ft 8in
Height	1.32m	4ft 4in

Capacity

Flight crew	1 / 2
Passenger seating	up to 11
Stretchers	1 stretcher + up to 7 medical attendants
	2 stretchers + up to 5 medical attendants

= Rotors turning

Maintenance and inspections

Specialist Aviation Services, the company that leases the AW169 to Dorset and Somerset Air Ambulance, has a team of engineers available round the clock to carry out maintenance on its fleet. Major inspections and overhauls of DSAA's AW169 take place after every 400 flying hours at the SAS base in Staverton, Gloucestershire. During that time a spare aircraft, an MD 902 Explorer, is provided for the air ambulance to use.

Routine maintenance is carried out at Henstridge Airfield by resident engineer Wayne Busby. He works a similar shift pattern to the crew, with four days on and four days off, and he aims to clear all upcoming maintenance for the four days he is away. If he isn't able to do that, or if something crops up when he is away or uncontactable, DSAA has standby engineers who come in, or SAS will send other engineers down from Gloucestershire. Wayne's main responsibilities are to forecast what might be coming up and arrange the spares or equipment necessary for a particular job. Depending on the nature of the maintenance, sometimes a second person is required to check his work, so he arranges for other engineers to come in and sign off. Initially it was expected that the AW169 would need an annual service, but as night flying has seen the number of flying hours increase, the first two years with Pegasus has been more maintenance-heavy, as lessons are learned about the new aircraft. As the aircraft matures, the frequency of services will probably be reduced and if DSAA can change its spare aircraft to an AW169, this will also make things easier.

On a day-to-day basis, pre-flight inspections are the responsibility of the pilot on shift, who has an extensive list of checks to carry out. Having first walked around and examined the general state of the aircraft's exterior, the pilot works through a checklist of things, including the security of the panels, integrity of the windows, hazards presented by any debris or unsecured items in the cabin or footwells, whether all lights are working, and if the gearbox area shows any sign of leaks. He will also look at oil levels in the gearbox and engine, examine the tail rotor for any damage and check for loose wires. Part of the inspection involves getting up to the head and spinning the blades, checking every blade for cracks or damage. The fuel tank is then checked for water, as is the 3,000-litre (660-gallon) fuel bowser.

A full system check of radios and navigation kit also has to be carried out once a day, as well as a power check of the engines. The aircraft has

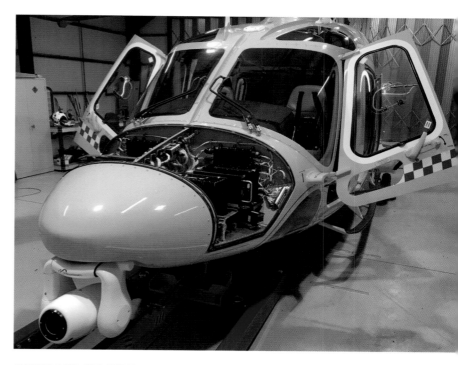

ABOVE AND BELOW *Pegasus* with its nose fairing removed, showing the 'brains' of the helicopter, as well as its navigation and auto-pilot computers. *(Wayne Busby)*

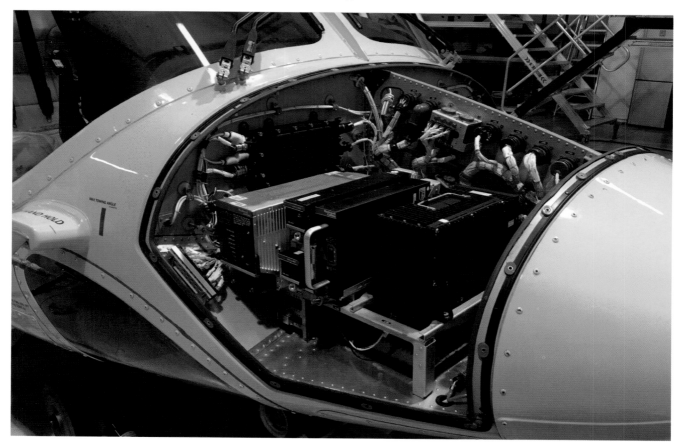

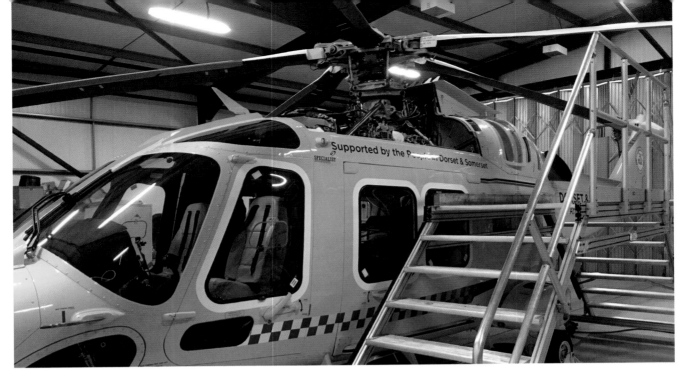

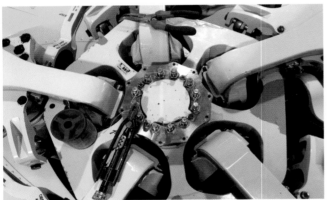

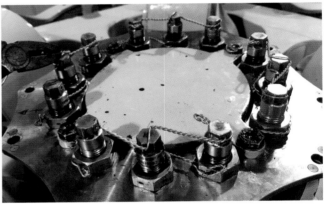

ABOVE AND LEFT The main rotor head and the lock plate that helps hold it on. Wayne recently had to remove the main rotor head to repair some damage before carrying out checks a few days later to ensure that the bolts hadn't lost their torque load once the helicopter had flown for a few hours. *(Wayne Busby)*

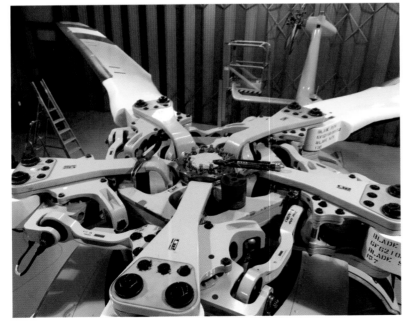

performance charts that let the crew know how the AW169 will perform in certain atmospheric temperature and pressure conditions. While the helicopter uses two engines to fly, it can manage on one for a brief period if one should fail. In order to be able to fly safely to a hospital, the aircraft has to have class 1 performance, which means that if at any point on the approach or take-off an engine fails, the other engine is good enough to allow the aircraft to either land or fly away.

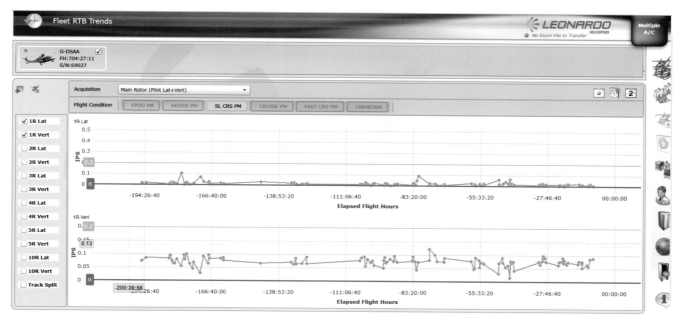

A daily power check is the only way to ensure that the engine meets this basic performance specification. Temperatures, pressure and speed of the engine are all checked and the data is put into a handheld device, which will tell the pilot the safety margin. This margin is constantly monitored to see if any dips occur that could signal a potential problem. If it dips below a certain level, the second engine wouldn't be able to cope, so the AW169 would not be able to land or fly away safely from the helipad.

ABOVE AND BELOW The Heliwise maintenance programme displays Health & Usage Monitoring System (HUMS) data that Wayne downloads from the aircraft. This data is the monitoring and recording of all of the component vibration levels in the aircraft, including the track and balance of the main and tail rotors. If the dots rise above the yellow or red threshold lines, or show a rising trend towards those lines, it is investigated and the necessary actions are carried out, either replacing, adjusting or rebalancing a component. *(Wayne Busby)*

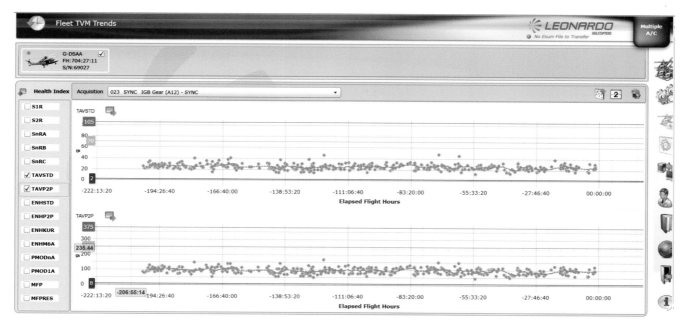

Wayne Busby is DSAA's dedicated engineer, working at the Henstridge base to maintain *Pegasus*. Wayne joined the army from school and did his apprenticeship as an aircraft mechanic, predominantly working with helicopters. He left the army after 14 years and worked as an aircraft mechanic with various companies before joining what was then Bond Air Services in 2005, where he started working on air ambulances. He worked firstly with Devon Air Ambulance, then moved on to Thames Valley for a year before joining DSAA when the previous engineer retired in 2014. When DSAA started operating the AW169, Wayne moved across from Bond Air Services to service provider Specialist Aviation Services so that he could remain with the DSAA team.

Generally working four days on, four days off, Wayne's main role is to manage all maintenance on *Pegasus*. His electronic maintenance programme shows all the scheduled maintenance on the aircraft, most of which needs to takes place after a certain number of flying hours, but some according to the calendar. Wayne uses his four days to try and clear the maintenance so that when he is away none will be required.

The AW169 large servicings are at 400-hour intervals. This aircraft flies between 400 and 500 hours a year, so bigger services come around every 10–12 months and are carried out at SAS's headquarters in Staverton.

With its night-flying capability, DSAA operates for longer hours than many other air ambulances, so its flying rate is higher. Planning ahead is important: during some periods of the year, such as school holidays, the Dorset and Somerset region is very popular with holidaymakers, so Wayne has to bear this in mind when scheduling the maintenance. 'I try not to impact on the aircraft's availability, so I tend to do lots of work early in the morning or late at night,' he explains. 'I try to leave it alone during peak times and at weekends, working around them to infringe on the crew's time as little as possible. They know that if I take the aircraft offline it's for a good reason, not for my own convenience.'

Should anything break down when Wayne is not on duty, he is available on the phone or via WhatsApp to talk the crew through any issues and is always within about an hour of where they are, so he can jump in the van and fix things if they can't be dealt with over the phone. If he is sick, on holiday or unexpectedly unavailable, there is another SAS engineer from a different county on call to clear unscheduled work.

Most of Wayne's duties involve dealing with routine problems and normal wear and tear on the aircraft. The sliding doors get a lot of use and can become stiff or sticky, so the rollers often need replacing or catches need fixing. The medical equipment, such as the moveable stretcher assembly, need keeping an eye on as they are also well used and if the mechanisms jam, the helicopter is useless for carrying patients. The AW169 has far more avionics than previous air ambulance helicopters, and occasionally things go wrong and there is no real explanation.

'I can plug my computer into the aircraft to interrogate it and find out what the problems are and whether they need urgent attention or can wait for software upgrades,' explains Wayne. 'Believe it or not, avionics systems are sometimes a bit like a home computer – you can often just turn them off and on again and that will fix the glitch.'

There are many shorter-interval scheduled

BELOW Wayne's engineer's log book and CAA maintenance engineer's licence, which authorises him to work on civil aircraft. *(Wayne Busby)*

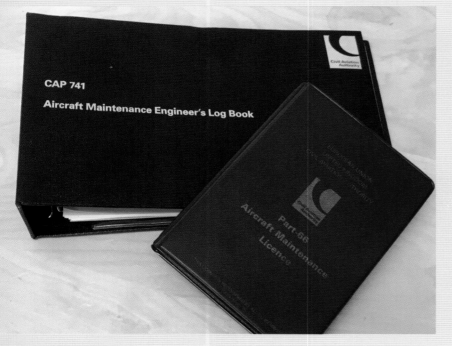

inspections to be carried out on the AW169, anywhere between 50 and 200 flying hours, as well as 30-day inspections. These are mainly visual inspections to monitor the condition of high-stress parts for wear and deterioration, such as components of the transmission, particularly the main and tail rotor.

Data from the engine and aircraft management computers are regularly downloaded to monitor operating parameters, any detected exceedances or anomalies, vibration levels and system conditions.

Keeping the aircraft looking spotless is also important, not only for its appearance in the public eye, but also because it makes it easier to spot any damage, wear or corrosion. So, Wayne can often be found touching up the paintwork and making sure the exterior is clean and shiny. Parts like windscreen wipers usually only need changing once a year and all the lights are LEDs, so bulbs no longer need to be replaced. Moving parts, such as the landing gear, are kept regularly lubricated.

Moving from the EC135 helicopter to the AW169 was quite a big change for all concerned. In engineering terms, the EC135 was a lot easier to maintain and in order to get up to speed on the AW169, Wayne was sent on a six-week approved manufacturer's course in Italy. The course, which is a CAA and

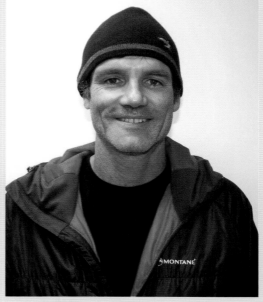

LEFT Engineer Wayne Busby is responsible for all routine maintenance of *Pegasus* at Henstridge Airfield.

EASA requirement, involved four weeks in the classroom and two weeks of practical work. While there, the engineers worked on prototype aircraft in the maintenance training facilities so they could gain hands-on experience, replacing parts and taking things apart. When he had completed the course, Wayne had to submit an application to the CAA through the compliance department of SAS, then wait to see whether the CAA granted him a type rating enabling him to work on the AW169. Had it been Wayne's

BELOW Wayne trained on the AW169 Maintenance Training Device at Leonardo Helicopters' 'A. Marchetti' Training Academy in Sesto Calende, Italy.
(Leonardo Helicopters)

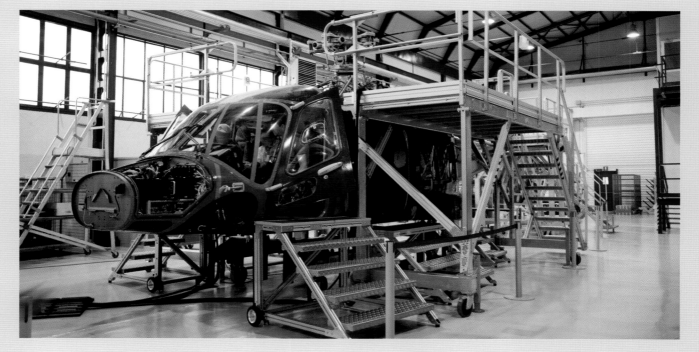

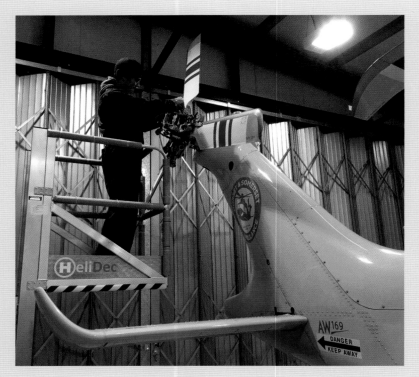

first time working on an aircraft, the CAA would require an additional six months of on-the-job training before Wayne would be licensed to work alone but because he has lots of prior experience and a range of helicopter types on his licence, he is qualified to work alone.

Aircraft engineers do not simply pass their exams and then keep their licences permanently. Wayne has to renew his type rating for the AW169 every two years, demonstrating that he has been regularly working on it. To do this, he keeps an engineer's log book where he records a broad selection of the jobs he performs, plus details of the work order numbers so that they can be checked by an auditor. He submits this through his compliance manager to the Civil Aviation Authority (CAA) so that they can check that his AW169 experience is current and his knowledge of the current EASA and CAA regulations are up to date. Also, Wayne has to renew his basic aircraft maintenance licence every five years, showing evidence that he has worked on aircraft for at least a six-month period in the last two years.

ABOVE Wayne at work on the tail rotor of *Pegasus*.

BELOW Maintenance forecast summary. *(Wayne Busby)*

Maintenance Forecast Summary

Specialist Aviation Services Ltd
21-Feb-19 W.Busby

Forecast In: **Hours**: 50	**Landings**: 200	**Days**: 30	**Forecast Date**: 23-Mar-19

G-DSAA	Helicopter, AW169	**TSN**: 833.25	**LSN**: 3094	**SRP**: 016/094622	**Flown**: 20-Feb-19

Aircraft

ATA	Ref No/Part No:	Description:	Serial No:	Position:	Alloc'd to Proj:	Hours Rem:	A/F Due Hours:	Cycles Rem:	A/F Due Ldgs:	Days Rem:	Date Due:	Compliance Within / Life Limits / Life Calculation:
32	32-38	Lubrication of the up/down lock actuator plunger of nose landing gear (NLG) and main landing gear (MLG) (Note 90)	69027			9.83	843.08		N/A	4	25-Feb-19	50 Hours, 30 Days
	50 Hour	AW169 50 Hour	69027			9.83	843.08		N/A			50 Hours
	50H 69027	50 Hour ICA 69027	69027			9.83	843.08		N/A			50 Hours
62	169-101	Service Bulletin SB169-101 Title ATA 62 - Damper Links Inspection	LK0298	Yellow		14.83	848.08		N/K			55 Hours
62	169-101	Service Bulletin SB169-101 Title ATA 62 - Damper Links Inspection	LK1189	Black		14.83	848.08		N/A			55 Hours
62	169-101	Service Bulletin SB169-101 Title ATA 62 - Damper Links Inspection	LK0446	Blue		14.83	848.08		N/A			55 Hours
62	169-101	Service Bulletin SB169-101 Title ATA 62 - Damper Links Inspection	LK0476	White		14.83	848.08		N/A			55 Hours
62	169-101	Service Bulletin SB169-101 Title ATA 62 - Damper Links Inspection	LK0656	Red		14.83	848.08		N/A			55 Hours
62	MI62-09	Main rotor damper link assy	69027			14.83	848.08		N/A			55 Hours
64	MI64-05	Tail rotor damper link	69027			14.83	848.08		N/A			55 Hours
79	PWC CU-001	PWC Oil Analysis Technology Trail Program	PCE-BP0056	Starboard		15.08	848.33		N/K			50 Hours
79	PWC CU-001	PWC Oil Analysis Technology Trail Program	PCE-BP0055	Port		15.08	848.33		N/K			50 Hours
62	CU169-005	MRH Sliding ring Re-grease	69027			17.17	850.42		N/A			40 Hours
64	MI64-04	Tail rotor damper	69027			21.83	855.08		N/A			62 Hours
56	PSEAW169/2018/9176 4/278243	PSEAW169/2018/91764/278243 G-DSAA Title: AW169 S/N 69027 (TT 755:35 FH, 2809 LDGs) – Lower Transparencies replacement deferral	69027			22.33	855.58	115	3209			100 Hours, 400 Landings
62	62-02	General Visual Inspection Of The Main Rotor Lag Damper Body	69027			22.33	855.58		N/A			100 Hours
67	67-16	Functional check (force measurement) of the collective pitch flight controls movement (Note 99)	69027			22.33	855.58		N/A			100 Hours
72	DAA2018-909-	DAA2018-909-PW210A-BP0055 Title:	PCE-BP0055	Port		23.24	856.50		N/K			100 Hours

BECOMING A TECHNICAL CREW MEMBER

EASA regulations mean that DSAA clinicians must obtain a Technical Crew Member (TCM) qualification in order to fly as part of the crew. SAS provides the necessary training package to bring the crew up to the right standard and Unit Chief Pilot Mario Carretta delivers the course at Henstridge, with the help of Pilot Dan Kitteridge.

Trainees go on a number of flights before undergoing a technical assessment, where they must demonstrate knowledge of aircraft safety, firefighting, navigation, communications and some of the basic functions of the helicopter, such as programming the navigation system, interpreting warnings and alarms and operating the windscreen wipers. Passing the course helps to improve the overall safety of the aircraft and its crew, as it provides TCMs with the ability to take on some of the basic cognitive tasks of the pilot, freeing him up to focus on more complex tasks.

Dan and Mario are responsible for ensuring that every crew member is a competent TCM and they carry out the final assessment and training flight, as well as additional or refresher training, should they deem it necessary.

Learning to fly the AW169

Commercial pilots are type rated, meaning that they are certified to fly individual aircraft types. They might be able to fly a number of aircraft within a category, perhaps two or three on the same licence, but whenever there is a change of aircraft, pilots must take a conversion course before they can fly the new one. Where that course is carried out is largely dictated by the complexity and maturity of the aircraft.

As the AW169 helicopter is relatively new, all pilots need to complete the manufacturer's conversion course, which is held at Leonardo's training academy in Sesto Calende, Italy. The academy is EASA approved and certified by the

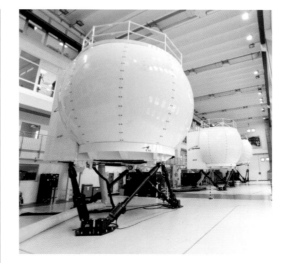

LEFT AND BELOW
The AW169 full flight simulator at Leonardo Helicopters' 'A. Marchetti' Training Academy in Sesto Calende, Italy.
(Leonardo Helicopters)

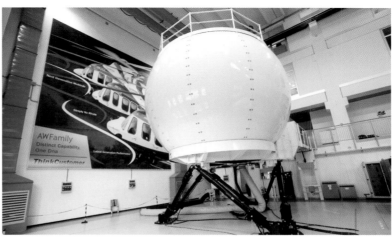

BELOW Each pilot undertakes around 30 hours on the simulator and, once the course is complete, spends a few hours flying the aircraft with an instructor.
(Leonardo Helicopters)

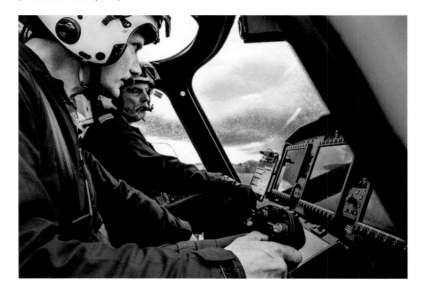

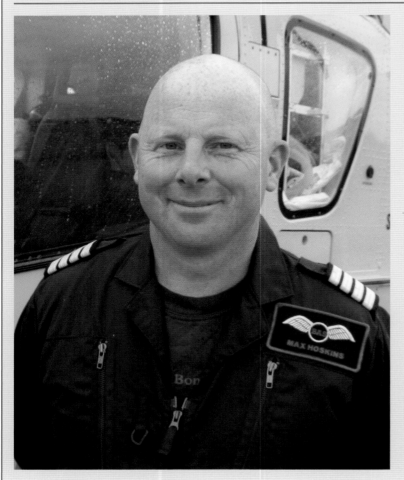

ABOVE Max Hoskins, DSAA pilot.

more variety. 'I have over 9,000 hours of flying under my belt now,' he explains. 'It would have been higher if I had stayed in the North Sea, but it's about the quality of flying not the quantity.'

In 2001, Max decided he would like to fly air ambulances, so joined Bond Air Services and embarked on a career as an air ambulance pilot, starting out with the Midlands Air Ambulance. During the past 18 years, Max has also flown Bölkows and EC135s.

'Back in the early days of air ambulances, no one had really thought about air ambulance helicopters in the UK, so you had to use what you had at the time,' he says. 'The Bölkow seemed to tick most of the boxes, as it was small and economical. It did the job at the time, even though you had to load the patient through the boot.'

During his time with DSAA, Max has landed on Glastonbury Tor, on beaches, on motorways and at the Glastonbury festival. He enjoys being able to think on his feet in a less structured environment. 'You don't know what you are going to every day and that uncertainty adds a bit of spice to the job.'

Dealing with the public is part and parcel of being an air ambulance pilot. 'The public love seeing us land, it's quite a spectacle,' says Max. 'I enjoy the show and tell element of it. You land and the clinicians go and do their job. Then crowds form and I am very happy to talk to them. I'm always mindful that these people are funding our operation. It all makes a difference, as people might see a collecting tin and put a few pounds in because they've just seen us that day.'

Like the rest of the DSAA team, it means a lot to Max when patients come to visit. 'When people come back to see us who are alive because of the air ambulance, that makes the difference,' he explains. 'It's also nice for them because when they last saw the helicopter they were probably in no fit state to appreciate it. And some of those who raise the most money for us are those we have previously saved or helped in some way.'

Max is the only one of DSAA's four pilots with a civilian background. He has been flying since 1986, when he started out with a private pilot's licence obtained through an RAF flying scholarship. He then tried flying helicopters and found he preferred them to fast jets, so got his helicopter licence in 1987. The following year, Bristow Helicopters sponsored candidates for commercial pilots' licences, so Max got his and then started working with them, flying all around the world to oil platforms.

Landing on moving decks and in atrocious weather in the North Sea is a very different sort of flying and after 13 years, Max decided it was time for a change. As a helicopter pilot, the main choices available to you are VIP work, search and rescue, or air ambulances and Max was looking for something with

Italian Civil Aviation Authority as an Approved Training Organisation. It has 18 dedicated classrooms and a maintenance training hangar, complete with two full systems trainers and full flight simulators.

The AW169 course runs six days a week, starting with ground school, where the pilots learn about the systems and the design of the aircraft in the classroom. After two weeks of that, each pilot sits an exam to make sure they have assimilated enough of the theoretical knowledge before moving to the practical element of the course. The practical lessons are simulator-based because the simulator is certified to such a high level that the pilots are able to carry out all training and exams using it. Each pilot undertakes around 30 hours on the simulator and, once the course is complete, spends a few hours flying the aircraft with an instructor.

When DSAA's AW169 is with SAS for repair or otherwise unavailable, the substitute aircraft is the MD 902 Explorer. DSAA's pilots also had to learn to fly this, completing an in-house training course with SAS instructors that took place about a month after they came back from Sesto Calende. No simulator was needed for this and the course was much easier, lasting only four days.

PILOT: PHIL MERRITT

When he was little, Phil wanted to be either a pilot, a fireman or a long-distance lorry driver. The lure of the skies proved too much and he joined the RAF straight from college, serving there for 19 years and undertaking tours with both the Army and the Royal Navy. When he left the RAF, he joined Bond Air Services as an air ambulance pilot, initially as a floating pilot covering various bases throughout the UK. As a Somerset resident, Phil was delighted when a vacancy came up at DSAA and he was able to join as a dedicated base pilot in 2008.

For Phil, the enjoyment of doing the job far outweighs the financial riches that could be had elsewhere and, like his fellow DSAA pilots, he thrives on the highly reactive nature of the work, never knowing what will happen from one shift to the next.

While the pilot's primary role is to take the clinical team where they need to be, Phil firmly believes that an air ambulance pilot should have the whole aviation package, not just the ability to fly. As the engineer isn't present at the base all the time, the pilot needs to be able to deal with the mechanical aspects of looking after the aircraft, including day-to-day duties such as refuelling, topping up oil, towing the aircraft in and out of the hangar, as well as performing all the necessary checks and preparing the aircraft for use.

Once he has flown the clinical team to an incident, he is also available to assist if

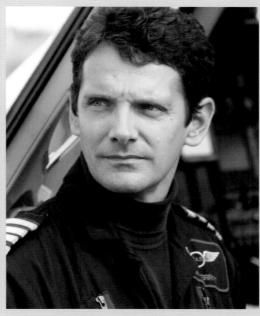

LEFT **Phil Merritt, DSAA pilot.**

need be. 'We can't leave the aircraft unless we can see it is completely secure,' he explains. 'However, if it is and we are not dealing with the public, we are very good at carrying bags or bringing specific pieces of equipment to the clinicians.' The pilots never touch the patients unless directly asked to do so, and they must remain focused on being able to fly the aircraft safely. 'If we became uncomfortable with any aspect of a medical situation, we would remove ourselves so that we don't see or hear anything upsetting,' says Phil. 'We mustn't be affected by the medical side of things so we must be able to switch off and remain detached.'

Chapter Four

The air ambulance in action

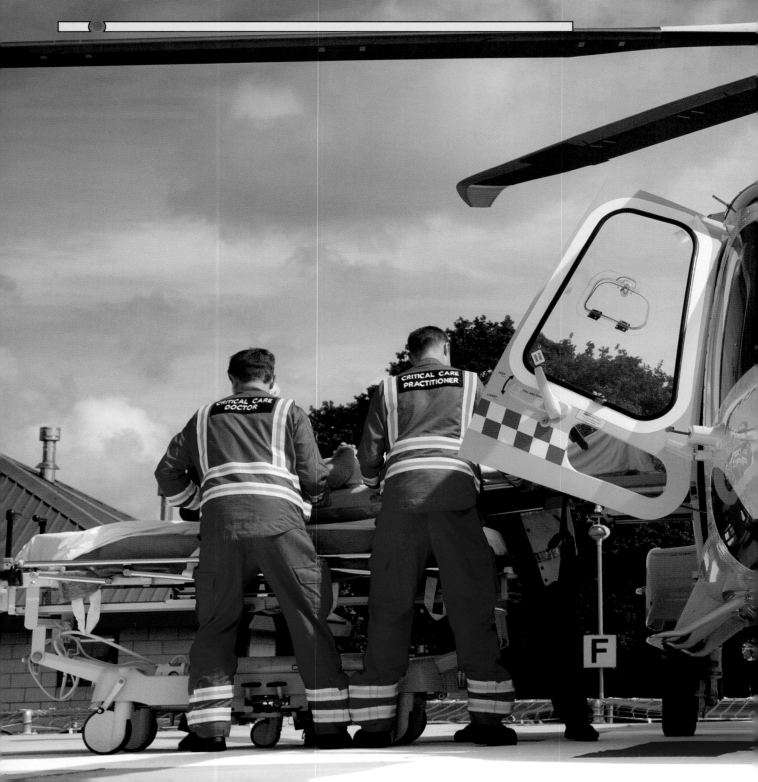

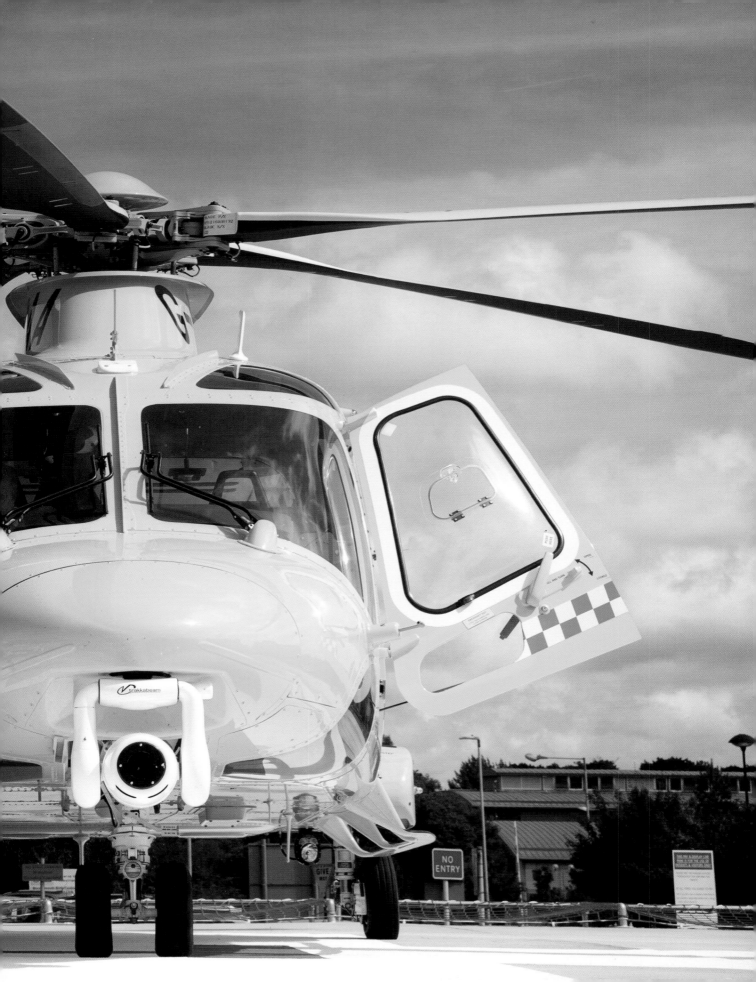

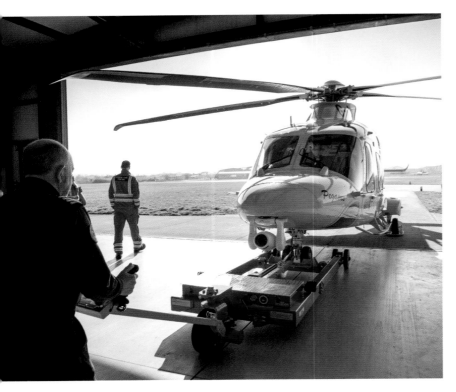

Mission timeline

As with every air ambulance crew working in the UK, no two days are the same. Once a shift begins, the duty crew can be tasked by the HEMS desk at any time to assist patients in any number of serious conditions in any location in Dorset, Somerset or even the surrounding counties. In order to operate the air ambulance safely and effectively there are rigorous checks and procedures that have to be carried out during every shift, with every crew member performing a vital role.

Pilot: arrival and preparation

The first shift of the day starts at 07.00h. When the pilot has arrived and changed into uniform, his first task will be to go to the office to check the paperwork on the aircraft and the notices to airmen (NOTAMS), which are notices filed with an aviation authority to warn of impending hazards or obstacles that may be nearby, such as air shows or cranes. The pilot will also check the weather, as climatic conditions such as temperature and pressure will affect the performance of the aircraft and the payload (weight it can carry) for that particular day. He then goes back to the

ABOVE, BELOW AND OPPOSITE TOP
An aircraft handling device is used to push the aircraft out of the hangar. The helicopter is connected up to the trolley-like device, which is then carefully driven out onto the tarmac. *(Simon Pryor)*

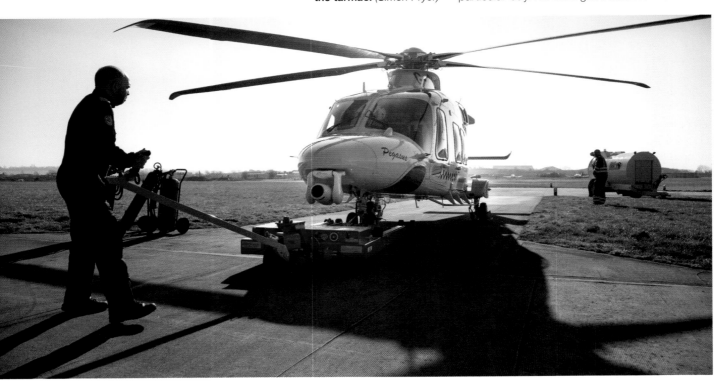

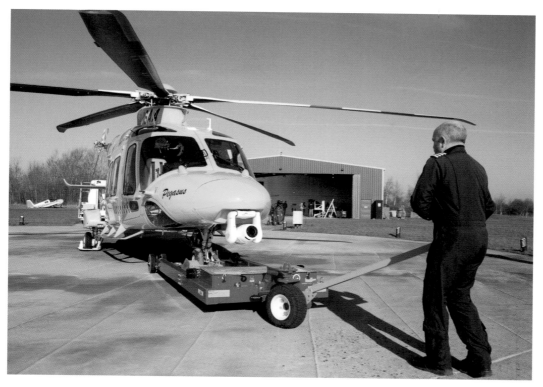

hangar and spends 20–25 minutes carrying out a thorough pre-flight check of the aircraft, opening up all the panels, checking the lights, performing a fuel check and draining some fuel out to check there is no water in the tanks. He will also check the integrity of windows, look for debris in the footwells or cabin and check the oil levels in the gearbox and engine, as well as inspecting the main and tail rotors for cracks or damage.

An aircraft handling device is then used to push the aircraft out of the hangar. The helicopter is connected up to the device, which is like a trolley, and it is then carefully driven out onto the tarmac, ensuring the blades don't hit anything. Fire extinguishers are then placed outside. From the moment it is unhooked, the helicopter is ready and a member of the clinical team phones the HEMS desk to say that the crew are online and ready to receive calls.

Pegasus's engines undergo a compressor wash every morning, where fresh water is put through the engine intakes. This is a requirement of the engine manufacturer as part of the warranty process. The starter motor is engaged to turn over all the turbine blades in the engine without igniting fuel, flushing the water through at the same time. This stops salt

and other contaminants from building up, which can affect the efficiency of the engine.

After the wash is complete, the pilot carries out a full ground run, which is a daily check of all systems. First, he starts the engines (drying

BELOW The AW169's engines undergo a compressor wash every morning, where fresh water is put through the engine intakes. *(Simon Pryor)*

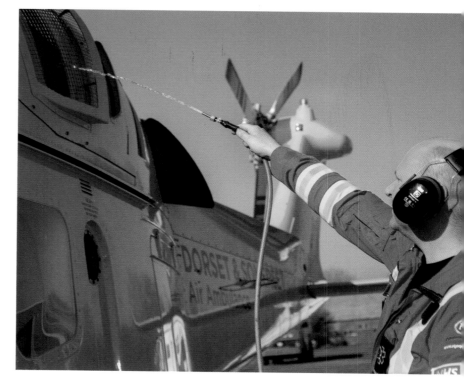

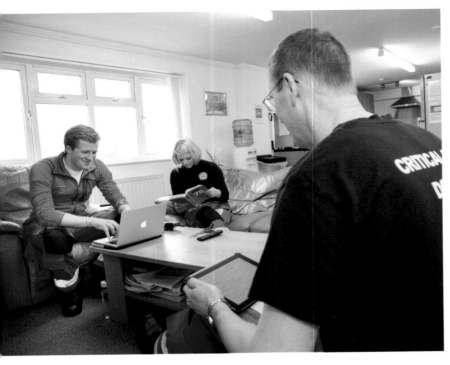

them out in the process). This also provides an opportunity to perform a power check, testing the power output from each engine separately to ensure they are performing at the appropriate power margins and working better than the manufacturer's minimum. To be allowed to fly to a hospital, the aircraft must have class 1 performance: should an engine fail at any point during approach or take off, the remaining engine must be good enough to allow the pilot to either land or fly safely away.

This data is entered into an iPad and then fed back to the Specialist Aviation Services (SAS) HQ at Staverton, so the company can keep an eye on the aircraft's performance. Should the performance start dropping off, the pilot would notify the engineer before it ever reaches the minimum requirement. If necessary, the engineer would then do a special chemical wash of the engines or carry out an investigation into why the performance is reduced.

Then it's time to join the clinical team for a formal briefing.

Critical care team: arrival and preparation

The clinical team arrives just before 07.00h and gets suited and booted while the pilot is carrying out his checks on the aircraft. They greet the pilot and then set about getting all the medical equipment ready. A clinical check of

ABOVE, RIGHT AND BELOW Critical Care Practitioners use a digital checklist to make sure all equipment is on board and all bags are packed. *(Simon Pryor)*

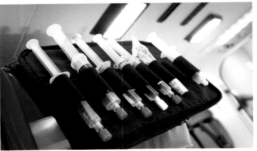

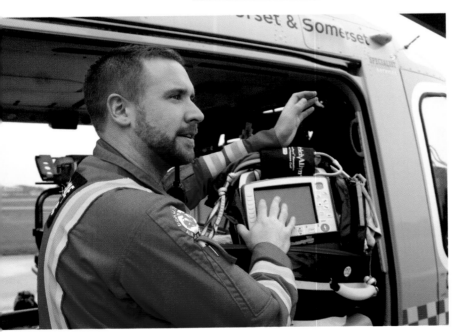

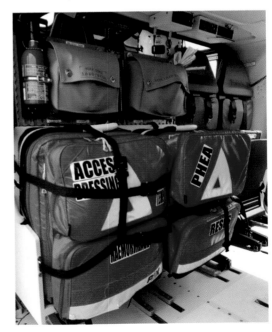

the aircraft is carried out, with the Critical Care Practitioners using a digital checklist to make sure all equipment is on board and all bags are packed, with everything sealed. Blood boxes and hi-visibility jackets are loaded into the cabin. The hangar doors are then opened and the clinicians help the pilot move the aircraft out of the hangar.

The AW169's payload is precise, so the crew have to weigh themselves from time to time, holding their helmet, jacket and flight suit. The pilot then inputs these weights into the relevant system so he knows how much payload is left – with the AW169, the payload is generous, so there is usually around 100kg (220lb) spare. These calculations are done first thing in the morning and again at shift changeover time.

Briefing and simulation

At this point, the crew try to have some breakfast, if they haven't already, as a call could come at any time and they have no idea when they will next have the opportunity to eat. Assuming no call has come through yet, the morning briefing then takes place from about 07.30h–08.00h and is a standard format, covering subjects from both the medical and aviation side of the operation. The crew assemble in the briefing room around the map table and go through a digital briefing sheet. Items on the briefing sheet include the weather, temperature, cloud base

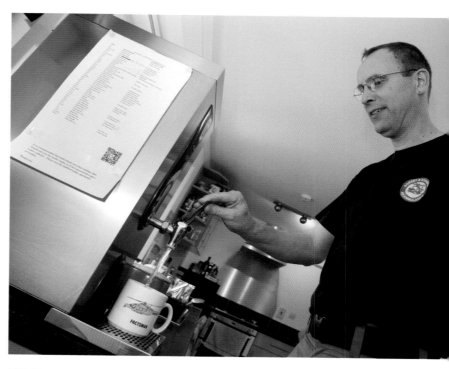

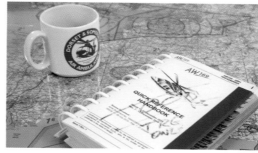

ABOVE Once everything is on board the aircraft, the crew try to have some breakfast as it may be a while until their next meal. *(Simon Pryor)*

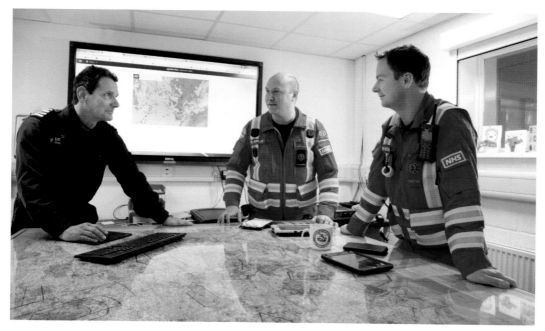

CENTRE AND LEFT The crew assembles in the briefing room around the map table to prepare for the shift ahead. *(Simon Pryor)*

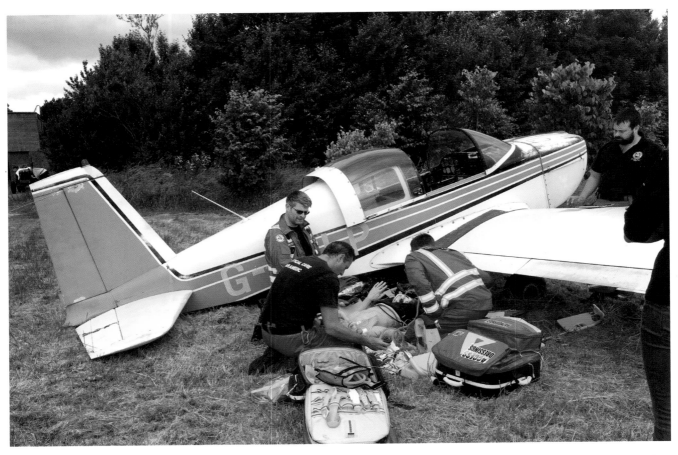

ABOVE The crew performs clinical simulations using props and manikins.

and NOTAMS, as well as things that have been published nationally about airspaces, restrictions to hospital landing sites and any unusual occurrences, such as thunderclouds. They also check when sunrise and sunset will occur and look at the diary to see what is happening around the airbase that day.

Adverse weather would be the main reason for DSAA having to turn down a job. Despite being an emergency medical service, the air ambulance is classed as commercial air transport by the Civil Aviation Authority, which brings a number of restrictions. For example, in order to fly, there must be a 500ft (150m) cloud base (1,200ft/365m at night) with 3km (1.9 miles) visibility.

Next, the clinicians decide who will sit where on the aircraft and then go through a complete clinical briefing, which includes equipment checks, battery checks, drug checks and finding out what sort of staffing is available from neighbouring air ambulance services. DSAA is the only air ambulance in the SWASFT region to carry a full critical care

team (including a doctor) day and night and it may be the only resource with a doctor in the peninsula at a specific time, so the crew need to be prepared for the fact that they may end up outside the counties' borders.

Once they have established that they are all well rested, healthy and fit to fly, the crew do a verbalised emergency run through of potential problems that may occur in-flight, using a randomised emergency machine that throws up a particular scenario, such as a fire in the engine. They also have emergency action cards to check that they have done the right thing.

The crew then performs a simulation of the day from a clinical point of view, using manikins to practise on. These manikins are state-of-the-art pieces of equipment that can be pre-programmed to display a set of symptoms – one of them moans and groans and its tongue can even swell up if required. Assuming no call has yet come in, the simulation usually takes place mid-morning and can either happen in the training room or outside. Depending on the simulation scenario, the crew can access other props such as a crashed aircraft fuselage and an off-the-road car.

The whole crew has a list of daily duties that need to be carried out. If time allows, the team also try to train every day and keep on top of their academic work, as well as carrying out any specific duties or responsibilities, such as checking and ordering drugs for the pharmacy.

Tasking and scrambling

When a call comes in from the HEMS desk, it comes through on a handheld phone with a specific ringtone. The team congregate in the operations room and there is an alarm to summon everyone from other areas of the base if they were not around to hear the phone. One of the clinical team takes the call and speaks to the HEMS dispatchers, based in Exeter. The dispatcher will give the crew a grid reference and these coordinates are entered into a tablet and also sent out to the pilot's tablet in the helicopter. The aim is to lift off within five minutes if possible.

By day, the pilot is given a location and, as long as the weather is fine and there are no hazards en route, that's all the information

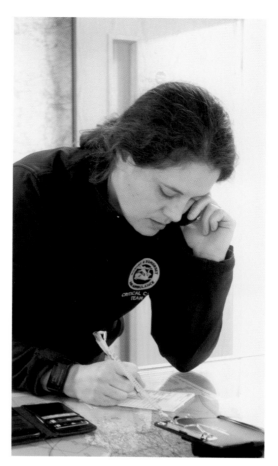

LEFT When a call comes in, one of the clinical team speaks to the HEMS dispatcher, who will provide a grid reference for the crew.

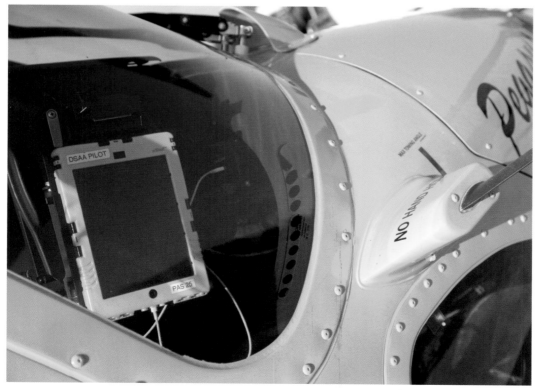

LEFT These coordinates are entered into a tablet and sent out to the pilot's tablet in the helicopter. *(Simon Pryor)*

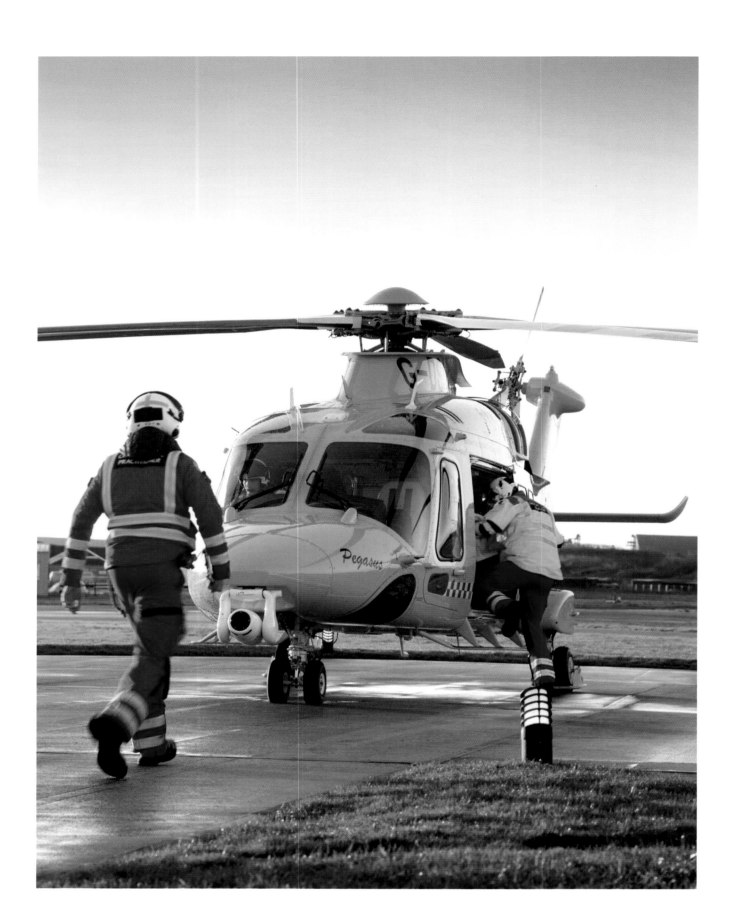

AIR AMBULANCE MANUAL

he needs at this point. This means that immediately after the call from the HEMS desk comes in, he can go and start up the aircraft while the clinicians are getting further details on the nature of the incident.

Despite the urgent nature of the call, all crew members walk out to the aircraft, rather than running. This is for a number of reasons, primarily safety, as they cannot afford to trip and injure themselves or damage their equipment. But it's also important that pilots and clinicians are in a calm, unflustered frame of mind in order to concentrate on the task at hand and perform their jobs properly, whether that involves flying to the scene or attending to the patient once they arrive.

Pre-flight

The tablets containing the coordinates allow the pilot to view maps at 50,000 magnification. During the day, he enters the grid reference and it converts to latitude and longitude, opening Google Earth so the pilot has a satellite view, which means he can see exactly what he will be dealing with in terms of fields, railway lines, roads and so on. Ideally, he will identify two

or three possible landing sites, in case any have been built on since the software was last updated. Another programme on the software shows power cables, but not telegraph cables. The software also marks sites where the helicopter has landed before and shows the accompanying notes made about it at the time. It also shows the nearest pre-reconnoitred site, so if need be, the helicopter can land there and wait for a lift from the police or ambulance service. These sites have all been reconnoitred by members of the team during the course of the year and are checked annually for changes.

Finding a landing site is just part of the job. It's also essential to check that the crew can leave the site quickly and safely. Google Street View is a useful tool for identifying openings and access points – there's not much point setting down in a field only to find there is no gate or that the exit is on the opposite side to where the crew needs to go. It can also help with spotting potentially hazardous wires.

The crew get into *Pegasus* and strap in. The pilot turns the power on, which gets the batteries up and running and all the internal computers booting up. While this is happening,

OPPOSITE The crew walks to the helicopter to avoid any risk of injury, rather than running. *(Simon Pryor)*

BELOW When finding a landing site close to the incident, it is essential to check that the crew can leave the site quickly and safely.

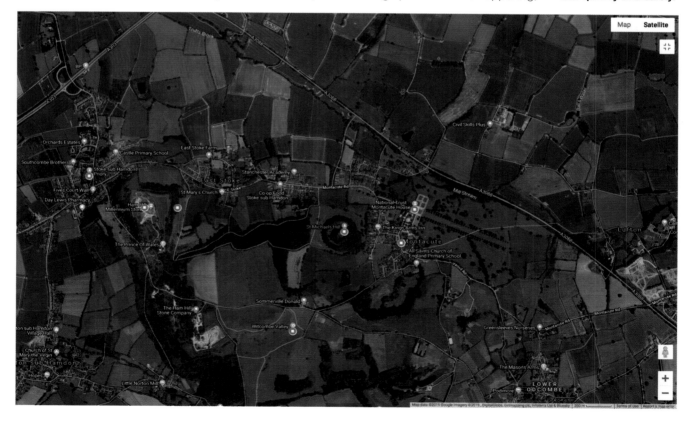

RIGHT The tablets containing the coordinates allow the pilot to view maps at 50,000 magnification.

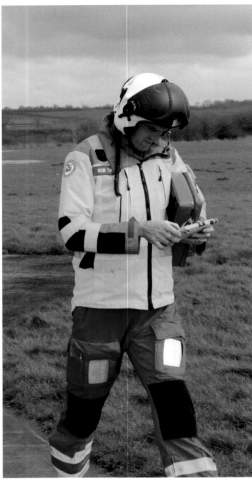

RIGHT The tablets containing the coordinates allow the pilot to view maps at 50,000 magnification.

BELOW During the flight the pilot and the Technical Crew Member (TCM) will listen to air traffic control, while the other crew member will take charge of radio communications with the control room, getting updates on the unfolding situation.

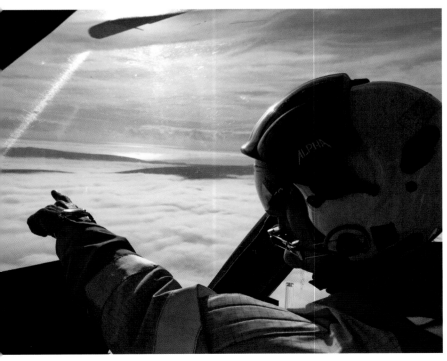

the pilot does a quick, final walk around *Pegasus* and checks that the doors are closed, looking at the general state of the aircraft. He then climbs back in and connects his helmet to the communications system to enable communication with the rest of the crew.

Having turned the fuel systems on, the pilot starts the first engine and the generator comes online to turn on the rest of the systems that haven't started up yet. He then starts the second engine, which starts the blades turning and brings them up to speed. A lot of the starting processes happen automatically, but the pilot and crew have to run through a series of pre-take-off checks to make sure everything is set up appropriately and in good working order to fly properly. Before take-off, the clinician who is acting as Technical Crew Member (TCM) will read out a challenge and response checklist to the pilot to ensure all aviation checks have been done and that all switches are in the right positions. They then read out another challenge and response checklist post-take-off.

The time between the tasking call from the HEMS desk and *Pegasus* lifting off is about five minutes.

In flight

During the mission, the pilot and the TCM in the front will be listening to air traffic control. In the back, the other crew member will ensure the equipment is safe and take charge of radio communications with the control room, getting updates and further clinical information on the unfolding situation. The crew is in contact with the HEMS desk at all times and the HEMS desk plots the helicopter's whereabouts.

Pegasus's call sign is Helimed 10 and when the pilot adds 'Alpha' on the end, it means the helicopter is on a job. Airspace is crowded in the UK and part of the pilot's role is to be in constant radio contact with an air traffic agency, so that if the aircraft does encounter a problem, he is able to tell someone where they are and what is happening. There are several cities in the region and if you are flying into a city's airspace, it's imperative to talk to air traffic control. Around Bristol, for example, air traffic control would ensure that charter flights avoid the route that *Pegasus* is taking. In Bournemouth and Bristol, it's often necessary

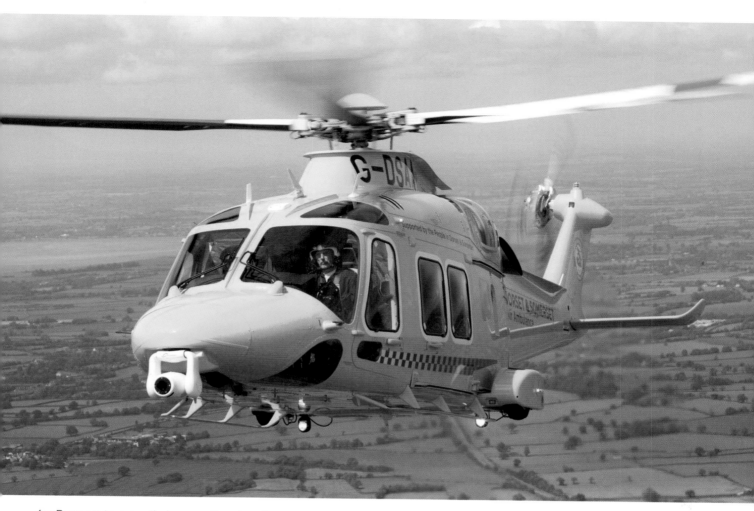

for *Pegasus* to cross their respective airport's runways, so air traffic control usually gets DSAA to fly over the centre of the field so that the big jets can still land and take off.

Landing

If the pilot hasn't had sufficient time to check the satellite images before take-off, he will instead observe from overhead and land as close as possible to where the patient is, orbiting the site once or twice to check for wires. During the day, an area of 30m (100ft) diameter is the minimum space in which the helicopter can land (60 x 30m at night) – there is a tool on the tablet that enables the pilot to measure a potential landing site in advance. Empty car parks can sometimes work, but they can also contain dangerous obstacles, such as concrete bollards. School playing fields or recreation grounds are often a safe bet. One of the pilot's priorities is not to damage people or

property: 'If we smash a car windscreen with a flying stone, we have failed,' explains Mario Carretta, Unit Chief Pilot.

If the pilot is unable to land the AW169 within 500m (0.3 miles) of the patient, the team would radio ahead and get a police car to meet them at the nearest landing site to convey the clinicians from there. The pilot would then remain with the aircraft and wait for a call on the radio letting him know what happens next, whether he is taking the patient onwards to a hospital or major trauma centre, or meeting the crew there because the patient is going by land ambulance.

Often a crowd will gather when *Pegasus* arrives and the pilot will find himself dealing with an interested audience. PR is part of the job and when people congregate around the aircraft, the pilots enjoy being able to chat to them while waiting for the medical crew. 'It's very humbling that people are interested in what we do,' says DSAA Pilot Dan Kitteridge. 'This is

ABOVE *Pegasus*'s call sign is Helimed 10 and when the pilot adds 'Alpha' on the end, it means the helicopter is on a job.
(Leonardo Helicopters/ Simon Pryor)

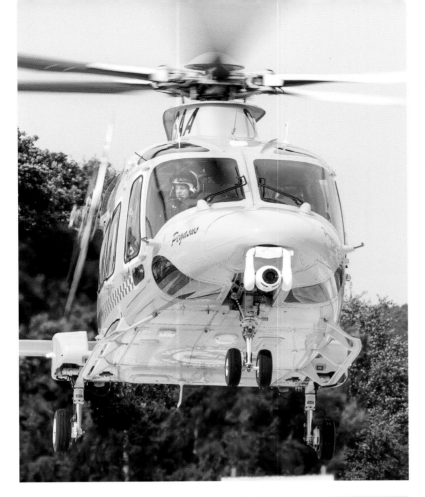

their aircraft, they fund it. If circumstances permit and we can show them how their money is used and the real effects it has, that's a very important part of the job. There are times when I have to ask for space as patients of course come first, but there are plenty of opportunities for us to be the interface between the charity and the public.'

If the patient is being airlifted to hospital, they are brought back to the helicopter and loaded onto the stretcher. Now that there are more landing sites, DSAA tends to visit big towns and cities more often than it used to and the team is lucky in that most major hospitals in their catchment area already have helipads: the two major trauma centres at Bristol and Southampton have them, as do the smaller hospitals at Taunton, Bournemouth and Dorchester.

As soon as the patient has been delivered to the hospital, the team is once again 'live'. The increased flying capability of the AW169 means that during the day, the team can retask immediately without going back to base.

Debrief

If no new job has come through, the team heads back to Henstridge, where their first priority is to ensure they are ready for the next mission. The aircraft is refuelled and cleaned, all the equipment is checked and the bags are restocked. Then the crew sit down and discuss the case they have just attended, from both a clinical and aviation perspective.

The aviation debrief is often more extensive at night because night flying is still relatively new and the crew are still learning. Sometimes they aren't able to land at the first site they selected, for example, so they would discuss why that was and whether people are happy with the fact that it had to change.

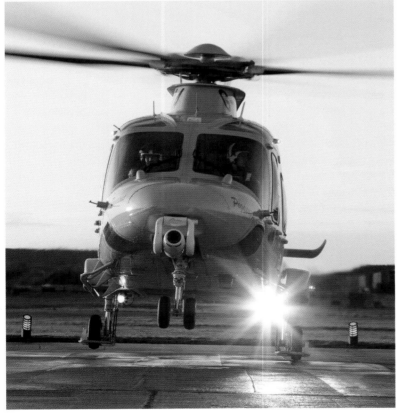

LEFT **Once the job is over, the team heads back to Henstridge to prepare for the next call.** *(Simon Pryor)*

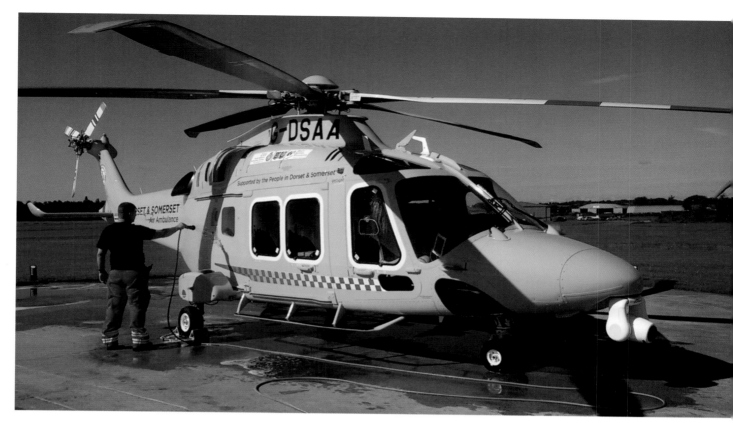

The clinicians also discuss the medical aspects of the incident, to check that everyone is happy with what happened. This involves following the patient's journey from the moment the crew arrived, to the interventions that were made and what the crew did before they left the scene or delivered the patient to hospital. Debriefs are currently ad hoc but the plan is to make them more structured in the near future.

Shift changeover

During the shift changeover period, the day crew and the late crew meet in the briefing room to complete a structured aviation and clinical handover. Clinicians change over at 16.00h and pilots at 17.00h, because pilots are only authorised to fly at night for a maximum of nine hours.

Any administration, equipment or vehicle issues are identified and if they have not been resolved, the late team take on the respective tasks. This also offers the day team a chance to update the late team on the incidents they have attended that shift and allows the opportunity for reflection and an informal debrief.

The late team get the night vision goggles (NVGs) and battery packs out, apply them to

ABOVE The aircraft is refuelled and cleaned in readiness for the next mission. *(Phil Merritt)*

BELOW During the shift changeover, a structured aviation and clinical handover takes place in the briefing room. *(Simon Pryor)*

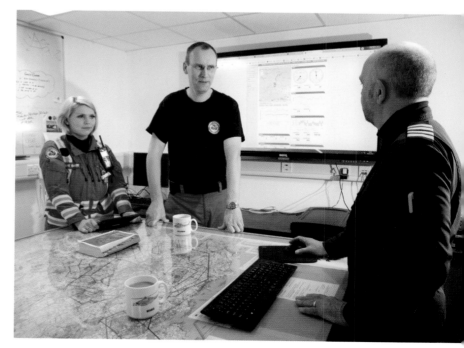

the flight helmets and set them up so they are mission ready. The team shares four sets of NVGs. When the duty crew sign out their set for the shift, the NVGs will probably have been used by someone else the previous night, and it is highly unlikely the settings are optimal for the new user. Using a Hoffman box, each crew member can set up their NVGs by looking through the letter-box opening on the box (while wearing the NVGs) and viewing a grid, which helps the crew member to focus the NVGs to their eyes. Once this is complete, the NVGs are ready for operational use as soon as a mission comes in.

End of shift

Towards the end of the late shift, the crew usually take out the towing equipment, connect it up and bring *Pegasus* back into the hangar. The bowser is locked and the fire extinguishers brought back in. The medical team give the inside of the helicopter a good clean, mopping out and vacuuming while the pilot performs his routine checks and preparations for the oncoming day. The clinicians turn off the oxygen and remove their medical equipment. The pilot puts the earthing cable onto the aircraft, gets the ground power unit in place and checks under the panels, so the aircraft is all ready for the morning inspection.

As the tyres on *Pegasus* are made from rubber, if any maintenance is done, static electricity could build up, which would cause damage to the avionics. The earthing wire means the aircraft is earthed, so this cannot happen. The ground power unit is essentially a big battery in a box, which can be connected to the mains and is used when the pilot or engineer wants to do maintenance or run checks on *Pegasus*, so they don't waste the aircraft's batteries. Before leaving the hangar, the pilot would also get the stepladder and staging out to put around the aircraft, saving the morning pilot from having to do it.

The NVGs and battery packs are removed from the flight helmets and locked away. The

BELOW Once the shift is over, the medical team cleans the inside of the helicopter while the pilot performs his routine checks and preparations for the next day. *(Simon Pryor)*

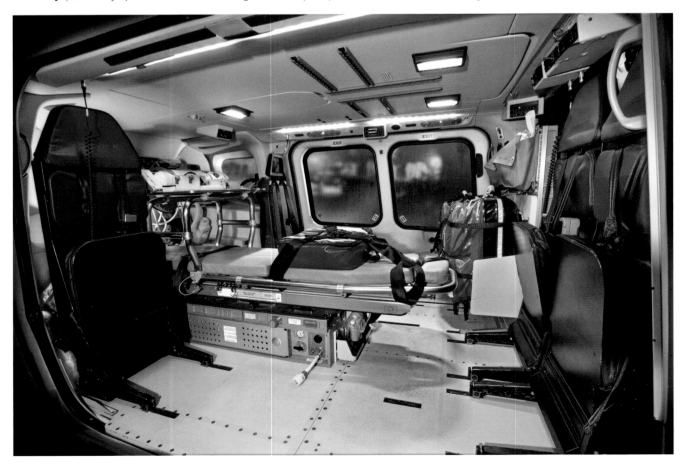

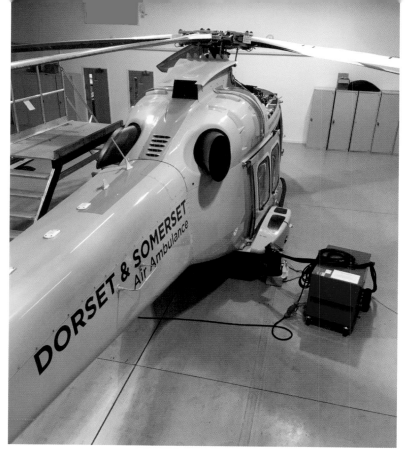

blood and drugs are signed back in and the radios and phone are put on charge. The crew makes sure the base is tidy and secure and then head upstairs to complete the final bits of paperwork. This includes completing the handover book, which informs the oncoming day team of any issues or tasks that may need doing. The pilot adds to the technical log, adding up the hours flown that shift. He prepares the next technical log sheet so it is ready for the morning, then puts any phones and tablets on recharge. Everyone then gets changed and heads for home.

BELOW Before leaving the hangar, the pilot puts out the stepladder and staging to save the morning pilot from having to do it. (Wayne Busby)

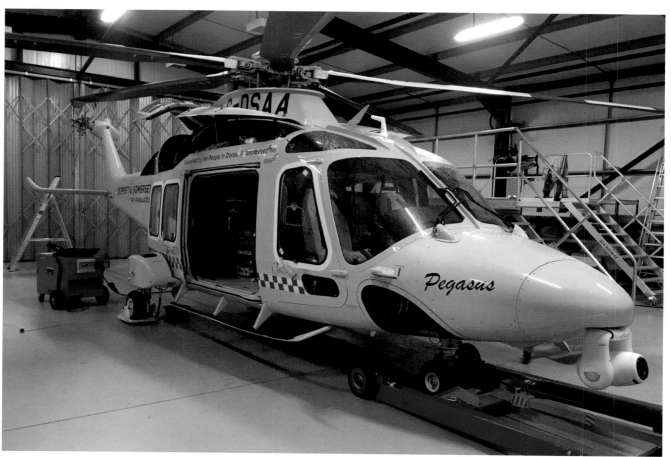

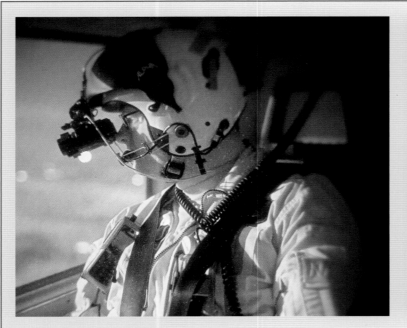

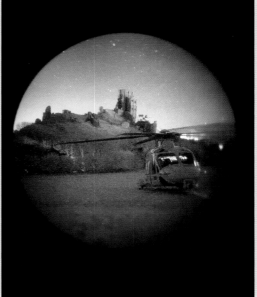

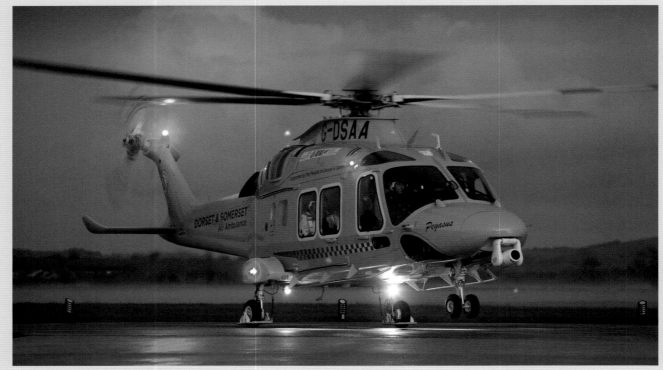

ABOVE At night, the team comprises one pilot, two CCPs and a doctor. The extra CCP acts as a Technical Crew Member, assisting the pilot.

NIGHT HEMS

When a call comes in during the hours of darkness, operating procedures are slightly different to those that occur during the day.

The aircraft is already outside, so the outgoing pilot hands over to the incoming pilot, briefing him on the weather and NOTAMS so that he can include that information in the team briefing. The pilot then gets out the night vision goggles (NVGs) and checks they are all set up correctly, placing them in the aircraft.

(Simon Pryor)

The crew all wear NVGs at night and also have handheld satnav capabilities and head torches. NVGs take in light and amplify it, but they need some light to work, so part of the evening briefing is to look at how much moonlight is expected that night.

At night, the entire crew must assemble in the operations room after the HEMS desk has tasked them with a mission. No matter how urgent the situation, the crew must undertake 10–15 minutes of planning before they can take off – and if they are retasked while out on a night mission they are only permitted to land at pre-reconnoitred sites, as it isn't possible to plan in the air during the hours of darkness.

At night, the DSAA team comprises one pilot, two Critical Care Practitioners (CCPs) and a doctor. An extra CCP flies with the crew at night and their main role is to act as a Technical Crew Member (TCM): supporting the pilot with navigation, reading out heights, speeds and rates of descent, as well as assisting with general awareness. They will also operate the Trakkabeam spotlight, which is situated on Pegasus's nose. Despite all the online checks, the crew will still do a recce around the perimeter of a landing site at night using the Trakkabeam to ensure there are no obstacles and they are happy to land. The Trakkabeam won't see wires, but it will pick up the posts that they are attached to. It's turned off before landing as the powerful light could damage people's eyes – the AW169's built-in landing lights are sufficient to get the helicopter on the ground.

DSAA is constantly looking at ways to improve the way it operates, both in terms of safety and efficiency. In consultation with the Civil Aviation Authority, it has now been agreed that lights will be installed along a section of the runway at Henstridge, allowing *Pegasus* to depart for an incident more quickly than it can from the helipad alone, and also allowing DSAA to use the runway at night. The charity will purchase the runway lighting and upgrade the current helipad lighting.

The patients

S ince it launched in 2000, DSAA has attended to thousands of patients across Dorset, Somerset and neighbouring counties. While DSAA is bound by rules of strict confidentiality when it comes to patients, a number of these individuals and their family members have been kind enough to share their stories with DSAA, for publication in the charity's biannual magazine and on its website.

Patient case studies
Maisie Sheridan
On 16 September 2016, 11-year-old Weymouth schoolgirl Maisie Sheridan was involved in a serious road traffic incident. A keen singer and dancer known for singing and performing at events in and around Dorset, Maisie was walking to dance class when she was hit by a van. Her mother, Ali, kindly shared her daughter's story.

'I had literally just walked in from work at 5.00pm when I received a call from my friend Mandy. Maisie walks to dance class every day with her daughter and friends. Mandy sounded panicky and then told me that Maisie had been

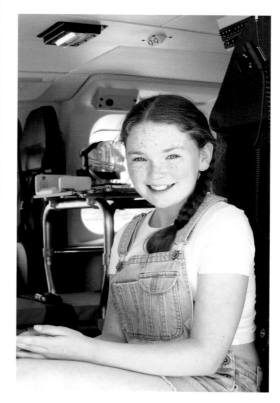

LEFT Weymouth schoolgirl Maisie Sheridan was hit by a van.

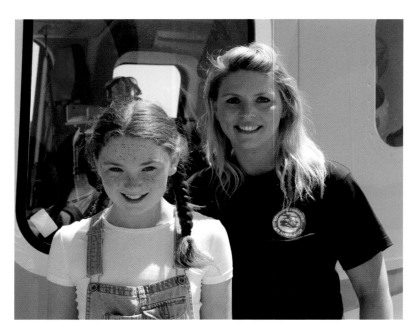

ABOVE Maisie Sheridan with Claire Baker, Critical Care Practitioner.

in an accident. My initial thought was that she'd fallen at dance class and at first I wasn't overly concerned. Mandy then explained that Maisie had in fact been struck by a camper van while attempting to cross the road. I went into overdrive: panic and fear. I jumped into the car with my other half Paul and rushed to the scene.

'Nothing could have prepared me for what I witnessed. The road was cordoned off and police, community first responders, an ambulance crew, an off-duty paramedic and passing first aiders were all attending to her.

'Maisie's face was badly swollen and she was thrashing around. The team believed that she could be suffering a brain trauma and had made a call for the air ambulance to attend.'

Pilot Phil Ware brought *Pegasus* in to land at a nearby marsh. The crew, Dr Rob Török and CCP Claire Baker, spent about an hour stabilising Maisie, who was put into an induced coma and prepared for an airlift to hospital.

'We were then driven to the air ambulance and secured in the aircraft,' Ali continues. 'Maisie was attended to and monitored throughout the journey to Southampton Hospital. At one point she began to vomit, but the crew swiftly cared for her and somehow, as frightened as I was, I knew she was being given the best possible chance of survival.

'The journey took approximately 20 minutes and when we arrived, consultants were waiting for her. She was immediately rushed to resus,

as time was of the essence. She underwent tests, which showed that she had fractured her skull and eye socket as well as having a couple of lesions on her brain. She had soft tissue damage to her groin and knee, and road burns to her torso. Due to the impact, Maisie also lost a layer of skin from her face – in her words, "I lost some of my freckles."

'Two days after the incident, Maisie woke up and asked, "Am I going to school today?" After four days she came home to recover and hasn't looked back. She begged me every day to let her return to school and her performing. She achieved great results in her first year back at school, and continues to sing and dance most nights. Thanks will never ever be enough and we are so grateful and lucky that the air ambulance came to her aid on that evening.'

As a way of saying thank you, Maisie has been fundraising for the charity by singing outside shops in Weymouth. Less than a year after her accident, she came to meet the crew who played a part in saving her life.

Shena Kozuba-Kozubska

Shena Kozuba-Kozubska lives in the small village of Donhead St Andrew near Shaftesbury and is well known nationally as an international horse trials competitor and trainer. On 11 August 2016, she had a serious riding accident while out exercising a young horse.

'I was two minutes out of the gate of my home when I pulled off the road to let a car pass,' says Shena. 'I remember turning to wave the car by, but that's it, no other recollection at all. Apparently one of the villagers was on his way to a funeral and found me lying in the road. No one saw what happened and we can only try and guess what the circumstances were; it may have been a noise, a dog or the car that frightened him. What is certain is that my injuries were extremely severe and possibly caused by the horse falling or trampling on me, although he had no signs of injury.'

The first thing Shena remembers is regaining consciousness in Salisbury District Hospital, four weeks later. She had been in intensive care in Southampton Hospital for two weeks and then spent a further two weeks in the intensive care high dependency unit at Salisbury District Hospital as it was closer to her home.

Shena then spent a further month on a ward. 'It was once I was transferred to the Clarendon Ward that my recovery really began,' she says. 'The staff were amazing and the ward is right on the edge of the most wonderful place, "Horatio's Garden". It's named after Horatio Chapple, who was the son of my surgeon and volunteered at the hospital in his school holidays. Tragically, at the age of 17, while on an adventure holiday, Horatio was killed by a polar bear.'

Having access to the garden to help with her rehabilitation was a key part of Shena's recovery. It is designed for people in wheelchairs and has an abundance of flowers that bloom at different times of the year. Shena was determined to get home, but the hospital wouldn't discharge her until she could walk up a very steep set of stairs to the spinal unit. Within two months of her accident, Shena managed to climb the stairs with the help of crutches.

'Although I think my recovery has taken ages, my doctors and physios are very pleased and almost astounded by the improvements I've made,' says Shena. 'Although I will not ride again, I am so lucky to be alive and still able to teach.'

Shena's injuries included a broken wrist, scapula and clavicle; left renal artery dissection; a subarachnoid bleed; a break to her left

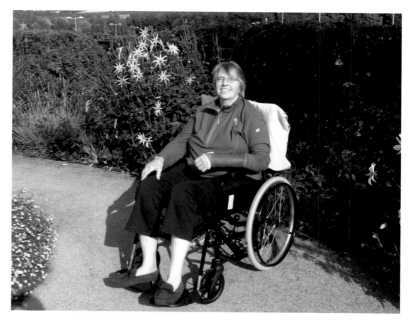

ABOVE Shena Kozuba-Kozubska had a serious horse-riding accident.

acetabulum (the socket of the hip joint), numerous breaks to her thoracic and lumbar spine; and an unstable L3 vertebra. She broke most of her ribs and suffered a bilateral flail chest (when a segment of the rib cage breaks due to trauma and becomes detached from the rest of the chest wall). She also suffered a haemopneumothorax (collapsed lung caused by air and blood leaking into the chest) and a pneumomediastinum (air leaking into the space

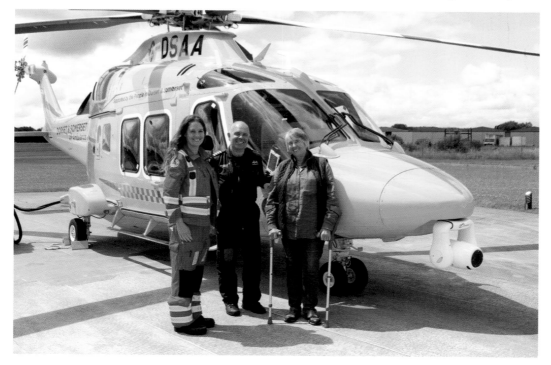

LEFT Shena Kozuba-Kozubska with DSAA crew members Mario Carretta and Michelle Walker.

between the two lungs, around the heart and the large vessels coming out of the heart).

'The work of the ambulance service paramedics and the air ambulance crew who came to my aid on that day was truly amazing,' says Shena. 'My goal is to hopefully gain a place in the London Marathon 2020 and run in aid of Dorset and Somerset Air Ambulance. Without them, I wouldn't be here.'

Ten months after coming out of hospital, Shena visited the airbase at Henstridge to meet Dr Rob Török, CCP Claire Baker and pilot Max Hoskins, who were working on the air ambulance that day.

Claire remembers Shena's accident quite clearly. 'When we arrived, our ambulance service colleagues were already on scene,' she explains. 'They had requested our assistance as Shena was likely to need critical care interventions and enhanced pain relief. When we got to her side, it was clear she was critically unwell with a broken arm and shoulder, many broken ribs and a life-threatening chest injury. She was conscious but in a lot of pain, so we administered a strong pain reliever, which also provided some sedation to help with her discomfort.

'The paramedic who had arrived on scene before us had put a needle into Shena's injured chest to prevent her lung collapsing. We now needed to advance her treatment, move her to the aircraft and get her to the right hospital as quickly as possible. We quickly gave her an anaesthetic and inserted a chest drain, which enabled us to take control of her breathing. This would give us immediate monitoring of both her lung inflation and developing chest injury.'

Shena was flown to the regional trauma hospital in Southampton, under anaesthetic. During the flight to the hospital, she became more unwell, with a drop in her blood pressure. 'This concerned us, as it meant that she could quite possibly have internal bleeding,' says Claire. 'In flight, we declared a "code red" to the hospital and on arrival were met by a large trauma team who were on standby with units of blood ready to administer.' DSAA now carries blood on board the aircraft and can administer it at the scene or during the flight to hospital, but in 2016 this service was not yet available.

After handing Shena over to the team in the emergency department, she received an immediate blood transfusion, a further assessment and a fast chest X-ray. The X-ray showed that a section of her fractured ribs at the back of her chest were pressing onto her heart, causing it not to beat as effectively. She was rushed straight to theatre where she had life-saving chest and abdominal surgery.

'It is amazing that Shena has made such a good recovery and was able to share her story and come back and visit us,' says Claire. 'She is a remarkable lady.'

Chris Pinnell

Good friends George Wiseman and Chris Pinnell are extremely keen cyclists. On 31 July 2016, a cycle ride on the Mendips ended with George helping to save his friend's life. Chris has no recollection of the incident, so George explains what happened:

'Chris and I had planned a fast and furious cycle ride on the Mendips with as many hills as we could cram in within our three-hour window. For the first time, Chris had agreed to take in a café stop around the halfway point. However, the events that unfolded that day meant we would never make it that far.

'After summiting Burrington Coombe, we proceeded along a well-cycled route towards Priddy. As we climbed to the top of a short steep hill, I became aware that Chris had dropped back. When I turned around, I saw him on the side of the road on all fours and in obvious pain. Very quickly, he collapsed, became unconscious and stopped breathing altogether. My military first-aid training kicked in. Fortunately another cyclist was in the vicinity and I asked him to call for an ambulance.

'For the next 20 exhausting minutes, while waiting for the arrival of the emergency services, I administered CPR in a bid to keep the precious oxygen pumping around Chris's heart and brain. Meanwhile, my ears were straining to hear the sound of not only a road ambulance siren but, given our isolated position, the sound of the whirling helicopter blades of the air ambulance.'

First to arrive was the land ambulance from Weston and local emergency medical Land Rover. A few minutes later, the air ambulance crew arrived and everyone worked together to try to stabilise Chris and prepare him for his flight to Bristol Royal Infirmary. He was placed on a stretcher and taken to the helicopter, having to be carried over a fence in the process.

'After 30 years in the military, I was well aware of the slick and professional teamwork of medical teams, but this was my first experience in a civilian setting,' says George.

The duty doctor that day was Rob Török, working alongside DSAA Operational Lead Paul Owen and Pilot Chris Whipp. 'We were tasked by HEMS control to a collapsed cyclist at 9:31 that morning,' says Rob. 'Within three minutes we were in the air on what was a bright and sunny day. We had a clear view of the ambulance and scene as we arrived overhead less than 20 minutes after our initial call. There was a suitable landing site just beyond the incident, with good access to the patient.

'The ambulance crew quickly provided us with an update on events so far, including the fact that they had already had to provide two shocks to defibrillate Chris's heart. I remember George confirming that he was trained and had provided CPR from the start of the incident as well as helping with information and logistics after we had taken over control of the situation.

'Paul Owen [DSAA Operational Lead] and I rapidly reassessed Chris's condition and we confirmed our plan to anaesthetise and intubate him. This was carried out before transferring him into the helicopter ready to fly to Bristol Royal Infirmary. Just as we were about to take off, Chris's heart once again stopped beating. After another defibrillation his condition remained stable throughout the 12-minute flight from scene to hospital. We then handed Chris's care over to the resuscitation team and cardiologist in the emergency department at BRI.'

Chris's positive outcome was most certainly due to a number of key factors. His initial difficulty was witnessed and responded to rapidly and effectively by a member of the public who had prior knowledge and training. An early 999 call was made to summon assistance and effective CPR was delivered by George until the ambulance crew arrived and took over.

Early identification of an abnormal heart rhythm was made, resulting in the provision of two defibrillation shocks followed by other

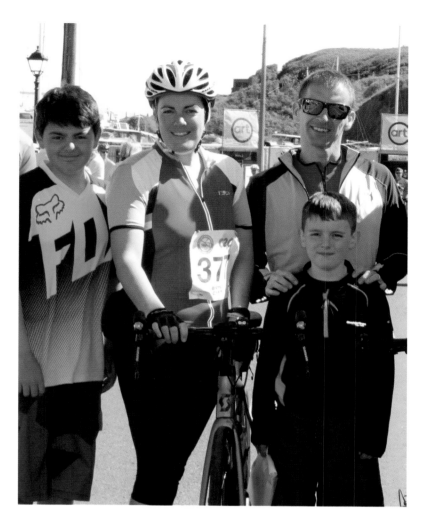

elements of advanced life support. Early tasking of DSAA's critical care team by the HEMS desk enabled specialist critical care skills to be brought to the scene and the helicopter enabled rapid transfer to the specialist hospital that would best meet Chris's needs.

Chris still has no memory of the incident. 'My brain blocked the events of what happened that day, although I was told that I reacted to George's voice at hospital. As a fit and healthy 46-year-old, who has exercised since being a teenager, never smoked, eats healthily and doesn't drink much alcohol, hearing that I had suffered a cardiac arrest was clearly a shock to me.

'After arriving at the Bristol Royal Infirmary Intensive Care Unit I underwent angioplasty (a procedure to widen narrowed or obstructed arteries or veins) and had two stents put into one of my arteries; I remained in an induced coma for the next 48 hours and when I awoke

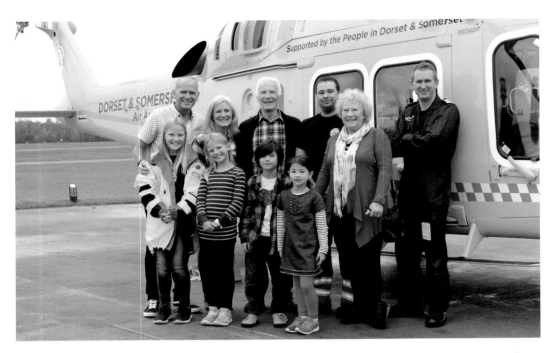

my wonderful wife was at my side and gave me the news.

'It is clear I owe my life to George, the NHS paramedics and, of course, the Dorset and Somerset Air Ambulance. It was certainly the intervention of the professionals that ensured I got to the hospital in excellent time and in a stable condition, which was critical to my survival.'

Like many other ex-patients, Chris, his wife and many of their friends and colleagues now support the charity.

David Little

David Little is a keen gym-goer and member of Gillingham's Fitness by Design. In March 2017,

while visiting the gym, David suffered a cardiac arrest and stopped breathing.

'The incident happened before I'd begun any exercise,' says David. 'I felt fine one minute and then suddenly collapsed while I was chatting to another gym member. Recalling anything after that is impossible, as my heart stopped beating and I was officially dead.'

Fortunately for David, the gym had a defibrillator and staff members undergo regular training sessions on its use. The defibrillator had been purchased in 2005 but this was the first time it had been used in real life.

The staff, together with the help of gym member Barbara Turnbull, who had 40 years of experience with the Red Cross, sprang into action. Personal trainer Ben Yorke began performing CPR while a colleague fetched the defibrillator. Together they worked incredibly hard to save David's life. CPR continued and the first defibrillator shock was given. Within four minutes the team had managed to restart David's heart.

Gym owner Colin Fricker was on hand with pure oxygen, which helped David until paramedics from the South Western Ambulance Service NHS Trust arrived. Due to the nature of the incident, the ambulance service called for the assistance of DSAA, who arrived in their rapid response vehicle. David was stabilised by Dr Phil Hyde and Critical Care Practitioners

BELOW David Little at Fitness by Design, with gym owner Colin Fricker, left, and PTs Charlie Patrick and Ben Yorke.
(Jane Norman)

Claire Baker and Owen Hammett before being transferred to hospital.

Every year, Dorset and Somerset Air Ambulance attends to numerous patients who have suffered cardiac arrests and the survivors of these events have all received early chest compressions and early defibrillation. When someone suffers a cardiac arrest out of hospital, if certain things are done in a particular order, that patient's chances of survival are greatly increased: this is known as the 'chain of survival'. The chain of survival consists of four links, three of which can be performed by any member of the public with basic life-saving ability:

1. Early recognition and call for help: the first step to helping someone who is having a cardiac arrest is to recognise that it is happening and call for assistance.
2. Early CPR: performing chest compressions can keep the patient's heart going until a defibrillator arrives.
3. Early defibrillation to restart the heart: early defibrillation can triple a person's chances of survival.
4. Post-resuscitation care: delivered by the emergency medical team who should arrive shortly after.

David's chain of survival was intact: he received immediate chest compressions, early defibrillation, post-resuscitation stabilisation and was transferred directly to a specialist heart hospital (which had the capability to perform the necessary procedures on his coronary arteries).

Following the crucially important chest compressions and defibrillation provided by the first responders, the DSAA team enabled David's heart and brain to be rested and for him to be safely moved, directly and rapidly, to the most appropriate hospital. Without any of these links in David's emergency treatment, he may not have survived.

'I spent eight days in Salisbury District Hospital, where I received superb care,' says David. 'I had three stents fitted and will need to take medication every day, but my GP has said that I should fully recover and be as fit and well as before.

'I have been told that only 10% of people who suffer a cardiac arrest outside of hospital survive,' he continues. 'I can only thank Fitness by Design owner Colin Fricker for having the foresight to have a defibrillator on-site and to everyone who helped save my life that day.'

David and his family have continued to stay in touch with the charity. During the half-term holidays, David and his wife Gill, together with their grandchildren, came to the airbase to meet the crew. He and Gill raised £1,400 when they asked guests to make a donation in lieu of giving presents at their golden anniversary party. These funds were shared between DSAA and the Stars Appeal at Salisbury District Hospital. David's daughter, Jen Rutherford, has also clocked up four half-marathons in aid of DSAA and more are planned.

Ben Yorke, the personal trainer at Fitness by Design who started David's CPR after he collapsed, was awarded '2017 Lifesaver of the Year' at the UK Heartsafe Awards.

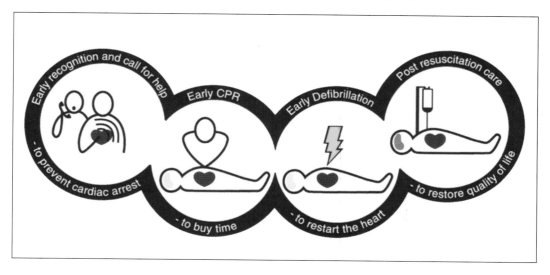

LEFT When someone suffers a cardiac arrest out of hospital, if certain things are done in a particular order, that patient's chances of survival are greatly increased: this is known as the 'chain of survival'.

Looking ahead

Much has changed in the air ambulance world since G-AZTI 'Tango India' took to the Cornish skies back in 1987. As documented in this book, in just over three decades the UK has seen air ambulance services launch right across the country, from the Orkneys to the Scillies. This growth has brought with it incredible developments in the capability of air ambulances in general, both in the diversity of the aircraft and road vehicles, and the individual skills of the crews concerned.

In the early days, no one had thought about adapting helicopters on the production line for the specific purpose of being air ambulances, so pilots and medical crews had fewer options in terms of which aircraft were available. Now, new helicopters are being designed and bespoke medical interiors are being created, with operators updating their fleets accordingly. These next-generation aircraft are far more advanced than their predecessors, using complex computer systems and offering enhanced reliability, safety and capability. Features such as autopilots and ground-proximity warning systems, as well as state-of-the-art medical interiors, are now commonplace.

These technological advances bring enormous benefits to patients, saving precious minutes when it comes to reaching them and offering enhanced treatment and care at the scene. This does come at a price: these larger and more complex helicopters are by their very nature more expensive to operate, while pilots need on-type training to fly any new aircraft. Increasing complexity and regulation also means that crews require enhanced training and simulation before they can take to the skies.

As we have seen, air ambulance operations in the UK have undergone tremendous technological advances in aviation but, just as significantly, incredible innovation in the clinical, pre-hospital area – underpinned by the General Medical Council's acceptance

of the new medical sub-specialty of Pre-Hospital Emergency Medicine (PHEM). Today's air ambulance crews are using increasingly sophisticated medical equipment, techniques and procedures, all of which require additional training and simulation, but undoubtedly provide a greatly improved service for patients.

At a national level, regulatory changes can have a profound effect on the way in which air ambulances operate. Since CAA regulations changed in 2012 to enable night-flying HEMS, for example, a large number of the UK's air ambulances are now flying during the hours of darkness. Some services are preparing to switch to 24/7 operations, while others are analysing the evidence to see whether round-the-clock operations are necessary in their own areas of the country.

Looking ahead, there is always the potential for political upheaval to impact on the way in which air ambulances are run. Currently, some air ambulance services are responsible for their own clinical governance, which requires them to

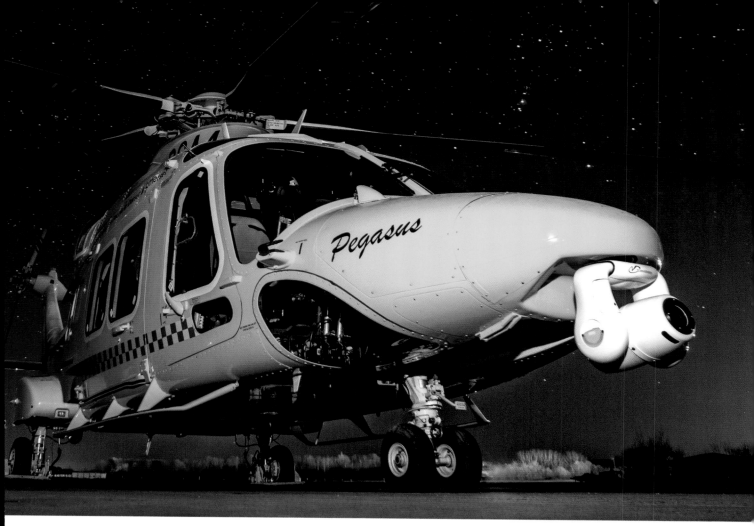

be registered with the Care Quality Commission (CQC), while others are clinically governed by their local Ambulance Service, and are not required to be independently registered. If the rules changed, preventing clinical governance being held by Ambulance Services on behalf of air ambulances, then all would need to be registered with CQC. Any changes to European Union Aviation Safety Agency rules could affect the way in which air ambulances are regulated in future, while global events such as recession would have financial consequences that could hit public purse-strings – and therefore the charitable sector – hard.

After 30-plus years, we are now moving into the second generation of air ambulance operation in the UK and no one quite knows what this will bring. Technological advances are a given, with enhanced materials, improved safety equipment and developments in helicopter avionics all increasing efficiency. Remote piloting and drones could start to play a part in reconnaissance. Telemedicine, where technology is used to deliver clinical care from a distance, could start to be a factor in the pre-hospital environment, enabling some patients to be examined remotely and allowing crews to send patient details digitally to the hospitals to which they will be transferred. We may see increased monitoring of flights for safety reasons, and greater use of technology when tasking aircraft – all of which has the potential to reduce human error throughout the whole system.

As night flying and 24/7 shifts see patient numbers increase, the already systemic approach to air ambulance operations will evolve and become even more effective, leading to improved tasking, closer working relationships with Ambulance Service colleagues, perhaps even a greater focus on prevention to help the public protect themselves. PHEM clinicians are at the cutting edge of medicine, developing new procedures all the time. For those patients across the country who may one day need the help of their local air ambulance, the future is bright.

ABOVE The UK's air ambulance helicopters provide an essential emergency medical service, but nonetheless rely on charitable donations to carry out their life-saving work. With continued support from both industry and the public, and the use of increasingly sophisticated technology, the dedicated teams that support and operate these services have a bright future ahead. *(Pete Appleby)*

Index